Diet Mindset Makeover

The Complete Guide to Repairing Your Relationship with Food

KARA BEUTEL, MS

ISBN: 1720590850
ISBN-13: 978-1720590859

CONTENTS

ACKNOWLEDGMENTS

First and foremost, I owe the deepest level of love and gratitude to my family: my husband, Brian; my son, Brandon; my parents, Tracy and Bruno; and my sister, Jenn. You each gave me your faith and support from day one, and I can't tell you how much I appreciate that. This book wouldn't exist without you all believing that I could do this. I love you all to the moon and back!

To my in-laws, Linda and Dieter, thank you for the countless hours you help by taking care of Brandon so that I can work. He adores his time with you, and I am grateful to have such loving and supportive in-laws!

To my mentor and friend Georgie Fear, I owe you a tremendous amount of thanks. Not only have I learned more from you than I did through all my many years of school, but your kindness, compassion, support, and guidance are worth their weight in gold. Thank you for being such a wonderful, sane, and trusted source in this industry, and for being such an amazing friend and mentor.

To Maryann Jacobsen, who helped to show me how to transform my course content into an actual book; thank you for your guidance and support. I wouldn't have even considered it possible to create this book without your suggestion. Thank you for the idea!

FOREWORD

By Georgie Fear, R.D.

Not all prisons have walls. In my years as a nutrition coach and clinical dietitian, I've interacted with thousands of people to discuss what they eat, and why. And many of them have been "locked up." Their confinement didn't begin with something as obvious or sudden as a door of bars slamming behind them. They usually don't know an exact date when it all began. But here they are, stuck. The "prison" of a diet mindset builds itself around you, and when you first notice these insulating thick walls, they can appear to be safety and protection.

Dieting can seem like it offers us a shield from becoming fat and ugly, and solace from feeling guilty or ashamed. A weight loss meal plan beckons to us as a refreshing oasis of organization amid the chaos of all the food decisions facing us. The promise of thinness is sold as a package deal of happiness, confidence, strength, and sex appeal. Of course we want those things; so we buy the magazine, print out the meal plan, or hand over our credit card to purchase 25 frozen meals without a clue as to whether they actually taste good.

There are enough solutions out there to keep us on this path for decades, tasting all the different flavors of the same thing. Whether we choose a points-counting diet, or dip into the cut-out-this-food-group diet, or try not eating at all for arbitrary segments of time, we are placing blocks in the walls of our diet mindset prison. Each block supports the others and the walls climb higher and higher. They all fit together, seamlessly, into a smooth surface of messaging that tells us we need rules from outside to correct us, contain us, and restrain us from wrecking ourselves with food.

Some people notice quickly that they are being deceived and they kick down the piles of blocks while they are just knee high. They stomp away, shaking off the dust, glad to have escaped with their freedom, and they don't look back.

I am not one of those people.

I let the walls of a diet mindset build and build throughout my youth, telling myself that I liked the shade, the coolness, and solitude I had inside. But when the day came that I thought it might be nice to explore what other people were enjoying outside, I could see no way out. I literally could not choose what to eat when I didn't have a system of externalized decision making. I needed to know how to dismantle the walls, and I needed direction to help me explore my life once I had the freedom to move again.

I found that leaving the diet mindset didn't mean giving up or settling for less of anything: it gave me greater health, a better performing body, more happiness with my appearance, more joy in food, and most importantly, more space in my life to get my head out of my abs and make a real difference in the world.

This book is your escape toolbox. In the chapters that follow, Kara walks you through the directions for taking down the walls and venturing back out into your life. The beautiful things that you want for yourself, like good health, happiness, and confidence, are *out there*--in the world, not inside the walls. There's a lot of exploring to be done once you're freed; plenty to engage a person for ten lifetimes, so there is no time to waste. Kara has put together an amazing and helpful resource; one you can count on and trust.

Let's get you out of your prison!

SECTION 1: THE HARMS OF DIETING

CHAPTER 1: WHY A DIET MINDSET NEEDS A MAKEOVER

I am so thrilled you've taken such a pivotal step toward repairing your relationship with food by picking up this book. If you're reading this, you most likely have been 'around the diet block' a few times. Whether you dieted to lose weight, to prevent gaining weight, to improve your general health, or to improve your athletic performance, somewhere along the way you started to pay attention to what you were eating.

That is a wonderful thing! Valuing your health and taking steps to take care of your body by feeding it well is something to be deeply proud of. Bringing a level of awareness and mindfulness to our eating is a powerful way to promote health. I just want to be sure that a critical point is brought front and center from the beginning: **There is a difference between *healthy eating* and *dieting*.**

Dieting Versus Healthy Eating

Dieting is typically done to lose weight. Of course, you can follow a specific diet for other reasons, like a medically restricted diet, or one which excludes allergens that could kill you. But by and large, most people start diets to lose weight or prevent gaining it. Dieting is a method to manipulate and control weight, *regardless of your actual health.*

Healthy eating, on the other hand, is something completely separate from the scale. It's a broader, more all-encompassing goal of wellness. It's about nourishing your body and caring for yourself, no matter what you weigh or how your food affects your weight. There are many benefits to improving your way of eating, besides the potential to lose excess weight. Focusing on healthy eating means we focus on all those health benefits, rather than on a scale number.

For most of us, diets were our introduction to changing our eating patterns. But most diets have some negative side effects:

- They reduce eating down into calories, macros (percentages of protein, carbohydrate, and fat), and points, essentially turning it into a math equation.

- They give you rules to follow, foods that are good or bad, allowed or forbidden.

- They cause you to worry about all the things that are bad for you and how everything you've done before has been 'wrong.'

- They make your weight the sole determination of progress.

- They call anything you do outside of the diet a 'cheat' or a failure.

There is so much mental anguish that comes along for the ride when we diet, and it ends up ruining our relationship with food.

Constantly dieting also keeps you in a perpetual state of working on your weight, rather than actually living life. It becomes all-consuming. Every food choice we make gets overanalyzed in terms of how it impacts your body or your compliance with the diet. There is no wiggle room, no flexibility for the fluidity that is real life. There is just rigidity. And rules. And fear-mongering. And guilt. And constantly starting over again and again. It's a vicious cycle.

The people selling us diets don't have our best interests (like our health) in mind. They just want to sell more diet shakes, protein bars, and restrictive meal plans. It's an entire industry built around making us feel bad about ourselves and our health so they can keep raking in billions of dollars in our perpetual pursuit of thinness.

They know that most diets fail and that theirs eventually will too. But they keep pushing it, because they know we'll continue getting frustrated and keep coming back to try again and again. They know that once we start dieting, we'll end up stuck in a diet cycle of being constantly on-again and off-again with diets.

The Diet Cycle Affects Us *and* Our Kids

When we have kids, the mental anguish and damaged food relationship we've built up over the years manifests into how we feed them. As parents, we want the best for our kids in pretty much every way. That, of course, includes doing our best to feed them well. We try to do so in a way that nourishes them, helps them to grow up healthy and strong, and fuels their nonstop activity level, all while making sure that we do what we can to prevent them from becoming overweight.

We are truly afraid of raising an overweight child. And that makes sense. Childhood obesity rates have skyrocketed. Health issues that were once considered adult-only problems such as high blood pressure, elevated cholesterol, and type 2 diabetes are now presenting in younger and younger children.

We want to spare our kids these health problems. But it's not just that. If we have ever been overweight ourselves, we know first-hand how cruel other people can be about weight. We know the comments and judgments that are given freely by others. We know how hard being large in a society that values thinness can be. For many of us, it's why we went on our own first diet in the first place!

Having gone through the diet cycle ourselves, we want to do everything in our power to prevent our kids from ever having (or wanting) to diet. We want to help them grow up with healthy habits and already having a healthy and happy relationship with food. We want them to enjoy eating like we used to, and not have to worry about their size or shape.

The Goal of This Makeover

In essence, we want for our kids what we didn't have. Somewhere along the way, we started to dislike our bodies and feel some level of shame for our size or shape. We decided we wanted to change ourselves, and that we were okay putting ourselves through miserable rules in the name of eating better. We figured it made sense to micro-manage our food and take the joy out of eating.

But not for our kids. We want better for them! Do you see the double standard? Let me tell you a little secret. Okay, it's not actually a secret... We deserve better too!

Through this book, you'll identify the areas where dieting has affected you. You'll find out what "brain worms" from your previous diets have lodged themselves in your mind, and how they influence your eating style today. You'll also see how the diet mindset you've developed plays a role in how you approach feeding your children, for better or worse.

Then, once we've taken stock of the diet mindset lingering inside, we'll work our makeover magic to deprogram that negativity right out of you. We'll repair *your* relationship with food so that you can guide your kids on that same path and help them develop that positive relationship from a young age. You will learn how to be the healthy role model you've always wanted to be.

CHAPTER 2: THE PROBLEMS WITH DIETING

Can you remember back to before you ever did any type of diet? If so, do you remember how you felt about eating? I don't know about you, but as a kid, eating was a totally carefree thing. I ate stuff that was yummy, played a bit, then ate something else that was yummy. That was it. I didn't have any thoughts of "This Pop Tart is going to make me fat," nor "Can you believe there's high fructose corn syrup in this ketchup?" I didn't analyze what percentage of "full" I was, or if I should include XYZ in my meal versus ABC. I just ate!

And I was happy. I lived life without a care in the world outside of whether or not I was enjoying my life. And that's the feeling we want to get back to, isn't it?

Kids do it rather intuitively. It's somewhere down the line that external factors start to ruin it. While we're adults now, and we've had the benefit (and sometimes misfortune) of many years of eating experience, we can learn a lot from our former kid-selves.

We may have more nutrition knowledge than we used to, but many times, that actually trips us up more than it helps. The internet is full of bad nutrition information, and it leaves most people more confused than enlightened. It only serves to bring us farther away from our happy and carefree eating roots.

Diets Take the Joy Out of Eating

But what if we decided to take back that joy? That is, of course, the overall goal of this mindset makeover... to take that joy back! When was the last time you were truly happy while on a diet? What about the last time you actually looked forward to the select few foods allowed on your diet plan?

I remember trying a diet plan with my sister back in the day, and if memory serves me right, we were roughly junior-high age (which makes current-me very sad). But the three-day diet told you exactly what to eat for each meal of the day. It didn't matter if you liked it or not, you had to eat what was planned for you.

And there was grapefruit in it. I absolutely hate grapefruit. I'm pretty sure I didn't even last the whole three days. It was miserable. And there are some very restrictive diets out there that are much longer than three days. That sounds like a recipe for frustration and anger in my book!

Suffering through food you don't like is actually the *least* of the problems with dieting, though. There are longer-lasting problems:

1. They don't work. We don't eat less, and we *gain* weight.
2. They ruin our relationship with food. We feel bad about ourselves, obsess about our food choices, and risk developing disordered eating patterns.

In a 2005 paper, the authors gave a beautiful overview of the controversy surrounding the idea of dieting:

> *"For normal-weight individuals, dieting is viewed as a major source of the rising prevalence of bona fide eating disorders and the spread of body dissatisfaction, binge eating, and extreme weight control practices among otherwise healthy normal-weight people (and young women, in particular). For overweight or obese individuals, dieting is viewed as ineffective in the long run, as generally incapable of overcoming biologically based determinants of body size, as lacking justification because the health risks of mild to moderate obesity are minor or nonexistent, and as generally creating more problems than it solves."[9]*

I can't think of a better way to put this entire issue into a short paragraph! In a world where we're fighting a true obesity epidemic, it's incredibly difficult to hear that dieting isn't working. But like with many important things, it's much more complex than just "it doesn't work, so stop doing it."

Why Doesn't Dieting Work?

Perhaps we need to be a bit clearer. Lowering calories to be less than a person needs to maintain their current weight *will* result in weight loss. That is a truth that can't be changed. When we say diets don't work, it's not that they don't decrease weight in the short-term, because they often do exactly that as long as we really are lowering our calories. The problem is sustainability: the weight doesn't stay lost. It comes back.

There are two main reasons for this problem:

1. **Why we do it:** Is our current weight truly a health risk and we'd do ourselves a tremendous benefit by losing weight? Or are we already a weight that's in the healthy range but we're unhappy about how it looks? These are very different reasons to focus on weight loss or dieting.

2. **How we do it**: There is a myriad of ways to decrease your caloric intake. Some ways are very strict, regimented, and difficult to sustain; other ways are more manageable. To put this in the simplest of ways: If it makes you irritable, stressed out and unhappy, you likely won't stick with it for long!

There is a lot of psychology that goes into the why and how behind our eating, which we'll cover as we go through this book. First, though, let's take a closer look at why diets don't work.

Being on a Diet Doesn't Mean You Eat Less

Fun fact: did you know that just because you consider yourself to be "on a diet" doesn't mean you eat less?

If the whole goal of dieting is to take in fewer calories, but we're not succeeding in doing that, then it's certainly not going to result in the outcome we're looking for! Several studies have shown that free-living people on diets, or who say they're "trying to lose weight" don't take in fewer calories than people who aren't dieting.[1-3]

That seems amazingly counterintuitive, doesn't it? How is it even possible to be on a diet and not lose weight? Are people just not trying hard enough or something?

This is where I think dieting becomes more of a mentality than an actual behavior: We *intend* to restrain our eating, but we have a hard time converting that intention into an *actual* decrease in our intake.[3]

I should mention that, in research, there are two types of dieters that are often lumped into one big group but have still been shown to be a bit different. If a person is purposely trying to lose weight through their eating changes, they are considered a "dieter." However, if someone is restraining their eating to prevent gaining weight, they are considered a "restrained eater."[4]

These two groups certainly have some overlap, since both of them are putting restrictions on their eating to a point, but the distinction should still be drawn. When the two groups are compared, dieters tend to experience more negative consequences than the restrained eaters.

In both dieters and restrained eaters, however, restricting their intake actually predicts future weight gain and obesity.[5] That's right. The more we diet and restrict our intake, the more likely we are to *gain* weight.[6,7]

While it's not yet clear why this is seen in studies, there are a few ideas: First, it's possible that a history of dieting and rebounding from diets causes a recurring theme of weight cycling, and the weight cycling is what causes ultimate weight gain. A second possibility is that those people with a tendency to gain weight are the ones often going on various diets and the diets are failing to prevent the weight gain from happening.[6] In either case, diets aren't helping, and people are ending up heavier than before the diets.

Wow. It is so disheartening to hear that all the effort and misery that goes into dieting isn't even helping us achieve anything! Either we are successful in the short term, only to rebound when we stop the diet, or we don't actually decrease our intake in the first place.

There is a deeper and more important issue with diets, though, and that is how they affect us mentally.

Diets Ruin Our Relationship with Food

If being on a diet doesn't mean we actually lower our intake, what does it mean? It means dieters worry more, and feel more guilt about their food choices. They obsess and think about food more often.[2,3,8] They also experience more intense and frequent food cravings.[3] People who diet are also more likely than non-dieters to develop "maladaptive eating behaviors" such as binge eating and emotional eating,[2] and even eating disorders later in life (as well as obesity).[7] In short: dieting makes us obsess about food.

But those consequences don't come from an actual caloric deficit. Instead, it appears they come from something called "perceived deprivation," a term that means "a psychological state of eating less than one wants." [9]

It's not that we're actually deprived of calories; it's the *perception* of not being able to eat the things around us that we want to eat.

So it comes back to the why and how, and the fact that most diets we've done in the past have served to instill a lot of food rules in us about what we "can" and "can't" have, coupled with these things being available constantly. This means we're constantly fighting ourselves over wanting something and feeling deprived when we "can't" have it.

By actively trying to restrict certain foods, dieters (and also restrained eaters) find those foods becoming more desirable. They think about, obsess, and crave those foods more often, and then when they're unsuccessful in restricting their intake, they feel guilty.[2,8,10] This guilt can negatively affect our eating patterns.

How? Let's take an example of something many people feel a bit torn about: chocolate cake. We love it, yet we fear it because we're told it's bad for us, or we believe we shouldn't eat it. Chocolate also happens to be one of the most craved foods.

"Chocolate-related guilt has been associated with self-reported dysfunctional eating patterns (e.g., restrained eating, emotional eating, bulimia), high anxiety, depression, low self-esteem, neuroticism, body dissatisfaction and drive for thinness."[11]

In a study that specifically looked at guilt or celebratory feelings about chocolate cake, the people who felt guilty about the cake reported feeling a lack of self-control and were less able to maintain their weight over a period of 18 months.[11]

Of the people in the study who were actively trying to lose weight, the ones who associated the cake with guilt *gained* weight, while the ones who associated it with celebration did not.[11]

That food guilt isn't doing us any favors, is it? It's causing us to engage in eating patterns we don't like, it makes us feel anxious and depressed, and it usually means we gain weight rather than lose it. All in all, dieting and feeling guilty about our food choices is robbing us of a happy and healthy relationship with food.

Where Does Eating-Related Guilt Come From?

Guilt is a feeling that develops when we betray one of our values or standards. When we realize that our actions or behaviors aren't in line with our intentions or goals, we feel guilty.

Now, most of us don't value dieting in and of itself. But we do seem to value being a certain weight, shape, or size. So when we eat something that we feel isn't going to help us get or stay this certain size, that's where the guilt comes in.

The question again is: Why? Why do we value thinness or smallness? We can blame society as a whole for that one. When society places a big emphasis on weight, appearance, and weight management, our feelings about food and eating become more negative. We start to move away from finding pleasure in eating and instead try to use it as a tool to achieve the weight or body shape that society deems appropriate or attractive.[2]

This focus means we end up more stressed, and enjoy our eating much less.[3] It also means that we start to feel bad about our bodies if we don't think they fit society's ideal standard. This body dissatisfaction that comes from internalizing society's standards as our own is what leads us down the path of dieting and subsequent disordered eating.

It's kind of easy to see how that can happen: Body dissatisfaction leads to diet/restriction, which leads to breaking the rules of the diet, which leads to feelings of guilt, which leads to disinhibited eating or bingeing.[5]

Diet/Guilt Cycle

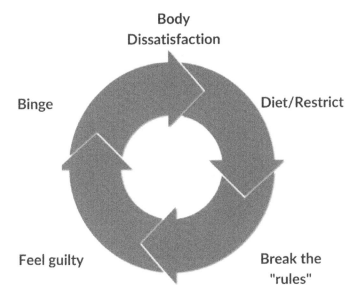

Do you want to know what's protective against the development of binge eating and other disordered eating patterns?

Self-confidence

This topic of body image, self-confidence, a focus on weight/size, and society's influence on the whole thing is such a fundamental part of this whole dieting equation that it makes up the entire next section of the book.

CHAPTER 3: HOW OUR DIETING AFFECTS OUR KIDS

Why is a Diet Mindset Makeover important for anyone but us? I'm so glad you asked. As parents, we are our children's primary role model. Your statements, actions, and general approach are being watched by the cutest little hawk eyes you've ever seen. Kids are taking everything in, and how *you* approach food and eating will shape how *they* approach it.

I love this quote from Ellyn Satter in her book *Your Child's Weight: Helping Without Harming*:

> *"Even if you only restrict your own eating, your kids are watching you. They will decide, 'when I grow up, that's how I will eat too.'"*[12]

That is both an encouraging and depressing thought. It's depressing because none of us want our kids to diet. We want to spare them that pain if possible! But it's also encouraging, because it means that if we can overhaul our diet mentality and practice the healthy and moderate approach to food that we want to have, our kids can start to learn that by example (without us having to try to drill it into them, because that's no fun for anyone!).

Think of How Your Actions Translate into Unspoken Words

Remember that old saying: "Actions speak louder than words"? It's certainly true when it comes to kids. Oddly enough, we can tell our kids things until we're blue in the face and they seem to not hear. But when they watch us do things or overhear the things we *don't* want them to hear (like curse words!) they somehow interpret that message *just fine*. They are watching and listening, and they're taking it all in.

Think about the messages that dieting and diet-like behaviors are sending to kids:

- Eating healthy is just to lose weight or be skinny.
- Being thin or skinny is the most important thing to be.
- You can only be happy if you lose weight or get thin/skinny.
- You can't trust your appetite or fullness feelings.
- How many calories (or sugar, or carbs, etc.) a food has determines if it's okay to eat or not.
- Certain foods are bad and should always be avoided.
- You're bad if you like and eat those bad foods, especially if you eat a lot of them.
- Being "fat" or overweight is the worst thing you can be.
- If you're overweight or large, people will make fun of you behind your back, or they may even "bully" you directly.

- Your body is not good enough as it is.

- Being on a diet is just something all grown-ups do and is totally normal.

- It's normal to think and talk about food *all* the time.

- Some foods can't be kept in the house because we can't be trusted around them.

- If we eat too much, we better work it off later at the gym.

Are these the messages we really want to send? Think about how you grew up. Did your own mother diet? How did it affect the way you relate to food and eating? Are there remnants of her mindset that you still carry with you?

As we'll cover more in-depth in the next chapter, one of the underlying reasons we diet is dissatisfaction with our bodies. By commenting negatively about your own body, kids learn that how your body looks is a vitally important thing and that being big, or large, or squishy, or fat, is "bad" or undesirable.

They start to take a look at their bodies in a way they never did before – in a way that says "I wonder what parts of *my* body are wrong and need to be 'fixed'?" This is where future dieters are created. Comments and actions from the most important people in kids' lives – their parents and family members – shape how they view themselves and the foods they eat.

Are You Ready for Some Sobering Statistics?

Kids are unhappy with their bodies from very young ages. Negative attitudes about body shape already exist in 3-5-year-olds.[13,14] By age 5, many children have started to internalize society's view of an ideal body size. In girls especially, this translates to a desire to be thinner by around age 6.[14,15]

"Body dissatisfaction is extremely common in preadolescence, affecting around 40% of children aged 6 to 11."[16] It affects as much as 70% of kids under age 6.[17]

According to the American Academy of Pediatrics (AAP), body dissatisfaction in teens is at about 50% of girls and 25% of boys.[18] (Yes, this affects boys too.) Body dissatisfaction has consistently been found to be associated with dieting and future weight control behaviors, including disordered eating.[16]

Even in teens who are of normal weight, about half of them are still unhappy with their bodies.[19] What is particularly upsetting is that this dissatisfaction with their bodies, the misperception of being overweight when weight is actually normal, and the resultant unhealthy weight control practices, all come together to result in many of these teens *becoming* overweight or obese in the future! This is true for boys as well as girls.[20,21]

Kids Are Already Dieting

It was mentioned previously that teens who are dissatisfied with their bodies tend to diet or use other unhealthy weight control practices, but unfortunately, it seems that dieting behaviors start even earlier than the teenage years.

Kids as young as 3-5 years old have been shown to have a basic understanding of the fact that eating less or moving more can help someone to become thinner, with 20-30% of 5-year-olds saying changes in eating or physical activity can be used to reduce body size.[22]

Not only do kids know eating and movement changes can change weight and size, but they also engage in actual dieting behaviors!

"Dieting in children is widespread with up to a third of 5-year-old children reporting engaging in dieting related behaviours."[22]

"Fifty percent of girls and 33% of boys have wanted to be thinner, and 40% and 24%, respectively, have attempted to lose weight."[23]

Different studies cite different rates of dieting in child populations. The Alliance for Eating Disorders Awareness states that almost half of 9- to 11-year-olds are "sometimes" or "very often" on diets. The parents or family members of these children are mostly on-and-off dieters too (82% of them![24]).

"In the 2011 Youth Risk Behavior Survey... 61% of girls and 32% of boys reported trying to lose weight; 12% of adolescents reported fasting, 5% reported using diet pills, and 4% reported self-induced vomiting or laxative use for the purpose of weight control."[25,26]

From the American Academy of Pediatrics paper on adolescents and eating disorders (emphasis mine):

*"Dieting, defined as caloric restriction with the goal of weight loss, is a risk factor for both obesity and EDs [eating disorders]. In a large prospective cohort study in 9- to 14-year-olds (N = 16,882) followed for 2 years, **dieting was associated with greater weight gain and increased rates of binge eating***

in both boys and girls. Similarly, in a prospective observational study in 2,516 adolescents enrolled in Project Eating Among Teens (Project EAT) followed for 5 years, dieting behaviors were associated with a twofold increased risk of becoming overweight and a 1.5-fold increased risk of binge eating at 5-year follow-up, after adjusting for weight status at baseline. Stice, et al. showed that **girls *without* obesity who dieted in the ninth grade were 3 times more likely to be overweight in the 12th grade compared with nondieters.** *These findings and others suggest that dieting is counterproductive to weight-management efforts. Dieting also can predispose to EDs. In a large prospective cohort study in students 14 to 15 years of age followed for 3 years, dieting was the most important predictor of a developing ED.* **Students who severely restricted their energy intake and skipped meals were 18 times more likely to develop an ED than those who did not diet;** *those who dieted at a moderate level had a fivefold increased risk."[18]*

Why Are So Many Young Children Dieting?

While it's hard to establish direct cause and effect, it has been shown that one important factor in the development of body dissatisfaction in young kids is parental influence.[17] Young girls (ages 5-7) model their mother's self-talk regarding body satisfaction. If mom is unhappy with her body, her daughter tends to view her own body in a negative light as well.[14]

Adolescent girls are more likely to be unhappy about their bodies and their weight if their mom is concerned with her own weight.[27]

Girls are more likely to diet before age 11 if their moms diet.[28] Forty-five percent of girls say their own moms "pushed them" to diet. Fifty-eight percent have been teased about weight by family members. This teasing is associated with higher body weight, unhealthy weight control practices, and binge eating in girls.[29]

When mothers directly mention a daughter's weight or encourage weight loss, it has a profound effect: "even subtle maternal encouragement, via mere mention of daughter weight, predicts young adolescent girls' greater dieting and lower body esteem."[30]

"Research evidence indicates that family-related factors are the strongest correlates of weight-related outcomes in children and adolescents."[31] This is the case in both positive and negative instances.

"Research studies have also demonstrated that parental weight-related attitudes and behaviors, such as weight-based teasing, weight and body talk, and parental modeling of dieting and unhealthy weight control behaviors are predictive of an increased risk of adolescent's engagement in dieting, unhealthy and extreme weight-control behaviors and binge eating."[31]

Well, That's Depressing! But There Is Good News Too

I don't know about you, but these statistics scare and sadden me. That's not the life most of us envision for our kids when they're born, is it?

We want so intensely to shelter our kids from being overweight that they're dieting and feeling badly about their bodies at younger and younger ages. That early dieting only leads to them gaining more weight along the way, resulting in the very thing we are trying to avoid!

For this reason, it is so critically important for us to develop a healthy relationship with food for ourselves, so that we can help instill it into them as well. After all, having a parent – especially a mom – who diets and focuses on her weight, means children are more likely to be dissatisfied with their bodies and engage in unhealthy weight control behaviors.

Some examples of things that promote a diet mentality or body dissatisfaction in our kids:

- Talking negatively about our weight, or theirs
- Talking negatively about anyone's shape or size
- Calling anyone (yourself included) names having to do with size (fatty, chubby, skinny-minny, etc.)
- Commenting on people's bodies (even complimentary, which I'll cover in the next chapter)
- Promoting certain foods as better than others, or healthier or "good for you"
- Telling kids that certain foods are "bad" or "not good" for them
- Restricting foods or keeping certain foods off-limits
- Talking about how many calories, carbs, sugar, or fat is in something
- Talking about losing weight or going on a diet
- Talking about exercise as a way to work off something you ate

Now, I realize that we all do some (or many) of these things. Don't worry; you didn't ruin your child for life. Until we start to see some of the research on kids and dieting, we are not aware that these things are being seen, heard, and internalized by our kids. So now that you know they're taking it all in, you can take steps to prevent talking this way in front of, or to, your kids. And no one is perfect at this, by the way! Even though I know these things, I still catch myself sometimes saying things along the lines of certain foods being healthy while others aren't. The point is to be mindful of it, and try to reframe things where possible.

There is good news here too. Just as kids pick up on our negative food/body talk, they also pick up on the positive stuff! We can set a healthy example and prevent dieting and body dissatisfaction in our kids by making simple changes to how we speak and act around food.

"Parents have the opportunity to positively influence their child's weight status through role modeling of healthful eating and physical activity behaviors, provision of healthful food choices within the home environment, and establishment of family norms around consistent meal and snack patterns, including regular and frequent consumption of family meals."[31]

It comes back to setting a great example, which I know we all strive to do in all areas of life with our kids! We model good manners so they'll pick up on them, we model good hygiene, and how to do chores. We can also model a happy and content relationship with food. But we don't want to put on a mask and pretend like we have this positive food relationship when we really don't. We want to enjoy that positive relationship with food for real! And so that's where this book comes in – to help you get there.

Learning to Set a Healthy Example

This change is not about finding the "perfect" way to eat healthily, or the secret to shielding our kids from our dieting adventures (like 'successfully' hiding our binges by doing them when the kids are sleeping). This is about getting the whole family to develop a generally sane, practical, healthy-without-being-dogmatic approach to food and eating.

To do that, we need to rewire that diet brain. It's been there for a long time, and it will likely put up a fight. But we can do this. We can pierce through all the fear-mongering and misleading info we've gathered over the years, and come back to a peaceful and enjoyable way of eating that both nourishes us and makes us happy.

Before moving on to the next chapter, I encourage you to take some time to reflect on your own diet mentality... the specific thoughts you have relating to foods, especially in terms of them being 'good' or 'bad,' the way you feel about certain social occasions that involve food, the way you feel about your body, etc. Taking stock of those things now will help you to make the most of this book, since it will allow you to see the areas where your diet mindset emerges, and the specific things that apply to your situation as you go through this book.

SECTION 2: BODY IMAGE

CHAPTER 4: NEGATIVE BODY IMAGE IS THE REASON WE DIET

Where Does Our Negative Body Image Come From?

Did you know that your negative body image thoughts aren't even yours? That sounds like a ridiculous statement, but stay with me on this one. When you were a kid, you probably didn't even think twice about your body. You just existed, and played, and ran around, and did whatever you thought was fun. You had no reason to think negatively about yourself until someone else planted that seed.

Maybe you have a specific person in your life who made comments they shouldn't have. That is, unfortunately, the case for some of us. But not everyone has a specific person they can call out as having put that very first negative body thought in their minds. For many of us, it's not a definite moment or comment that caused a turning point. Rather, it is the gradual build-up of various societal and marketing messages that we started to take to heart.

As women, we have been conditioned to think lowly of ourselves. Every single advertisement you see for makeup, shampoo, razors, clothes, and even yogurt, is geared toward making us feel like the way we currently look isn't good enough. Everything is marketed to us, as women, to 'fix' something about ourselves to make us better or more attractive. Forget that!

Think about it for a moment. Have you ever noticed just how many things get marketed to us by preying on the fact that we do not love ourselves?

- Have thin eyebrows? We've got a pencil to 'fix' that.

- Have laugh lines (from a life full of joy I might add)? We've got the Botox to 'fix' that.

- Have cellulite like pretty much every other woman on the planet? We've got a cream to 'fix' that too.

We Are Always Being Told We Are Not Good Enough

"If tomorrow, women woke up and decided they really liked their bodies, just think how many industries would go out of business."
– Dr. Gail Dines

I adore that quote because it so simply drives home the point that pretty much every industry is out to make us feel bad about ourselves to get us to buy their products. It's not just make-up, clothes, and other beauty supplies, though. One of the biggest problematic industries for how we view ourselves is the diet industry.

Diets try to convince us that there are tons of things we need to fix about ourselves and our eating. They tell us how our current stomach is too big, so we have to flatten it, or they tell us that we need their magical system to achieve the elusive thigh-gap. They tell us our current way of eating is 'toxic' and makes us store fat. They tell us that we're not attractive or lovable if we're not an ultra-thin runway model.

All of this messaging only serves to make us feel bad about ourselves and how we eat. We are living in a constant state of being told to be better because who we are now isn't enough. And we have internalized that message so deeply that it's become part of who we are. I'll say it again: Forget that! We can learn to eat well without believing that we are just one big walking bag of problems that need fixing.

We Are Being Told to Value Thinness

Not only is the world around us making us believe we have various problems to fix, but everywhere we turn people are also instilling a narrative that thinness and beauty are more important than everything else. Society is telling us to value being thin over being happy, or successful, or intelligent, or hard-working, or brave, or funny, or talented.

What is the one thing every single famous woman gets comments about in one way or another? Her appearance. It doesn't matter if she's a politician, actress, athlete, activist, entrepreneur, or performer. Her talents and attributes play second fiddle to how she looks and what shape her body is in.

Media and society have drilled into us that there is only one ideal standard of beautiful: a thin, shapely woman. This is what gets plastered on every magazine cover, every movie poster, every girl's toy, every *everything*!

We are all holding ourselves to an impossible standard. And it ends up leading us to feeling a deep dislike, or even hatred of our own body. We feel that our body is not as good as those cover model bodies simply because it is different, and we start to get sad and angry about that. Combine this unrealistic ideal with the constant messaging that we need diets, expensive make-up, and Botox to fix ourselves, and we have a recipe for self-disdain. This is body dissatisfaction; and this dissatisfaction leads the vast majority of women to feel like they *should* be on a diet or *should* be losing weight as we engage in the never-ending pursuit of looking like a cover model.

We need to start paying more attention to how often our body image is preyed upon. Not everything is about losing dress sizes, having the most luxurious eyelashes, or receiving the admiration of men. Our bodies are not billboards; they are our own personal business. It's high time we start to take our power back and start to tune out the negative messaging from all around us.

Your Current Body Deserves Love

The first step in reclaiming our power is to realize that *we* are the ones who get to say how we feel about ourselves. Not society, not the media, not the airbrushed swimsuit models. *Us.* We have to start challenging the narrative and changing the view we have of ourselves.

- It's not okay to look in the mirror and pinch our "flabby" spots and tell ourselves how gross we look.

- It's not okay to look at ourselves and think "I'd be so much prettier if ..."
- It's not okay to hop on the scale and have the number staring back at us dictate how we feel about ourselves that day.

We can do better. We can have better. And it starts with us. It doesn't matter if you are 100 pounds or 600 pounds, your body is worthy of love. You have spent your entire life in this body. It has been with you through tough times and good times. It is your physical presence on this Earth, that's all. The size and shape of your physical presence mean very little in the grand scheme of things. You, as a whole person, are valuable, lovable, and awe-inspiring, in whatever body you already have.

We are all different, in so many more ways than just outward appearances. There are things about you that set you apart from the crowd and make you unique. Your body is just *one* of the many things that make you who you are. We tend to put a disproportionate amount of our focus on how we look, what size clothes we wear, and what the scale says. But these are incredibly small pieces of the bigger picture, and they're rather unimportant! How you look doesn't make you who you are. At the risk of sounding too cliché, it's what's on the inside that matters most.

A Note about Being Postpartum

Since this book has several sections dedicated to how we influence our kids, it's a safe bet that many of those reading this are moms, and as a mom myself, I need to talk about something that is specific to us: We all have postpartum bodies. Whether we had our babies yesterday or 20 years ago, we have a body that previously carried a child.

If we didn't have body image difficulties before we got pregnant, chances are they started to come up after our bodies went through such a profound physical metamorphosis. I understand – I have been there. I remember being massively pregnant and wondering if I'd ever look like my former self again. I remember being newly postpartum, with a belly I still didn't recognize, and how weird that felt.

I also remember how, everywhere I turned, there seemed to be something advertising ways I could 'lose the baby weight' or 'get your pre-baby body back!' There were belly wraps, diets, special foods, workouts, and all sorts of products marketed exclusively to those most vulnerable of us – women who are swimming in a pool of intense emotions, in a body they barely recognize, who are sleep deprived, exhausted, and caring for a new human life. How absolutely obnoxious is that?!

There goes society again, telling us what we should be focusing on. Funny how what they think we should focus on is actually the *least* important thing going on at that particular moment of a woman's life. But that doesn't stop those messages from filtering deep into us. We've got about a million things going on when we first bring a new life into this world, and yet there is still some little piece of our brain space that starts thinking about losing the 'baby weight' and how our new body looks.

Don't let society tell you that you need to get back to a pre-baby weight or size or shape. You do not. All you 'need' to do is take care of your little one (even if they're big now!) and yourself. That is all. And that includes loving the body you have now, regardless of what it looks like, or how different it is from what you may have expected.

Our postpartum bodies are amazing. Yes, they've been stretched. Yes, they've been used as a nutrient delivery system. Yes, an entire person has exited our bodies. And those things only serve to make our bodies *more* amazing, not less. We will never get our pre-baby body back. We can't go back in time to before all those incredible things happened in, and to, our bodies. And that's 100% okay.

We are different now than we were before kids, in so many ways, not just in weight or size. We are moms now. And I don't know about you, but I am a better person because of it. Sure, I'm a more tired person, and a bit more stressed – always worrying about my little man and wondering if I'm doing a good job at this whole mom thing. But I am forever changed for the better.

Going back to my pre-baby body would mean that I didn't get the pleasure and privilege of knowing this incredible little human. And there is nothing in me that wants to go back to how things were before.

I have a very deep respect for what my body, and that of all other moms, has done. Many of us will carry the scars of our pregnancies and births for the rest of our lives. But they are battle scars to be immensely proud of. Without them, our kiddos wouldn't exist. Don't wish to erase the physical reminders of what you went through to bring them into this world. They are a part of the new, and even more awesome, you.

CHAPTER 5: CHANGING OUR FOCUS

Taking the Focus Off Looks

I read an article recently in which Renee Engeln, PhD, author of the book "Beauty Sick," was interviewed. I've not yet read the book itself, but it sounds like it falls right along this line of thinking that I'm discussing in this section. I pulled some noteworthy quotes from the article because the words are so powerful I couldn't possibly paraphrase them and still do them justice:

> *"Beauty sickness matters in part because it hurts,' Engeln writes. 'But even more important, it matters because **it's hard to change the world when you're so busy trying to change your body**, your skin, your hair and your clothes. It's difficult to engage with the state of the economy, the state of politics or the state of our education system if you're too busy worrying about the state of your muffin top, the state of your cellulite or the state of your makeup."[32]* [Emphasis mine]

How incredibly, and importantly, true is that statement?! I mean, really, that's the entire point of this section all wrapped up in one small paragraph!

How we look and what we weigh are such minuscule pieces of the grander picture of who we are and how we interact with the world we live in. Why do we give it such a disproportionate amount of our brain space?

We do it because of the conditioning I mentioned in the last chapter. And the author in the article mentions this too. She talks about how it's easy to get angry at society as a whole for instilling such appearance-focused negativity and judgment into us at every turn. But we can only control the things that are ours to control, and that starts with us:

> "Even though it's a cultural problem, the easiest behaviors to change are our own because we have so much more control over those," she said. "People say to me, 'We should fight the media!' Absolutely we should. **But we should also stop saying awful things about our own bodies in front of our daughters. And we can do that today. Right away, we can change our conversations.**"[32]

YES!! That is exactly what we're talking about here!

Should We Comment on Looks at All?

In the article, and I'm assuming also in the book, Engeln talks about not mentioning looks at all when speaking to or about other women.

Take a moment to think about just how hard that is to do. She's not just talking about judgmental or mean comments either, like saying awful things about our bodies or others'. She's also including compliments in that. Her approach is not to mention looks *at all*.

No telling someone they're pretty or that they have gorgeous hair (because why do those things matter?). It comes across as a bit of an extreme approach, at least to me, since I've always considered compliments to be a generally nice thing to say. I mean, if I don't know someone, and I notice something nice, why not tell her that I think she has fabulous hair, or that I'm impressed by how strong her arms look? The world is a very negative place these days, and compliments feel good!

But she mentions that even the nice compliments fuel the underlying narrative that women are supposed to look good, and usually that means society's version of "good." We are not put on this planet to look pretty. We are so much more than that! It's an interesting take on things, isn't it?

Finding Something Else to Comment On

I was thinking about this when an intriguing Facebook post came across my feed recently. The post, written by a man, was this:

> *"A woman updated her profile pic, like we all do. Five dozen comments about how hot, beautiful, sexy, pretty and gorgeous she is, all from other women. Never happens with men that I've seen. How strange it would be if I ever got five dozen men commenting on my looks from simply updating my profile pic... Makes me go hmmmmm."*

So true, right? I've noticed this a lot myself when friends update their photos and get a bunch of comments on their beauty. If we are all so much more than just our looks, why do we continue to focus on our looks?

The discussion that ensued from the post was really interesting. Some suggested that women are looking for compliments when they post pictures of themselves (my two cents on that one is that it's a profile picture— it's supposed to be of yourself!). Some people thought he was overthinking things and that the comments were just people being nice.

Other people talked about how they've started to notice this too, and how they've started to take on the approach of not commenting on friends' looks in their pictures. Instead, they comment about how the person seems to be feeling in the photo ("You seem so happy/in love/excited/etc.") or about the other aspects of the photo, like the gorgeous scenery on a vacation picture.

If we want to start taking the focus off looks, it has to start with us. And so I think the key takeaway from the above exchange is that we can start doing this by purposely trying to find something other than just a person's appearance to comment on, whenever we can.

An interesting follow-up to that friend's post happened a bit more recently too. He posted another observation along these same lines:

> *"Just saw a picture of a bunch of very attractive ladies. Not one comment about how beautiful they are. Why not, every picture of women gets a flood of other women commenting on their looks, why not these ladies? I wonder if it is because they are super successful and confident and their friend circle thinks that there are other things more interesting about them than their looks."*

Kind of drives home the point, doesn't it? There is so much more to comment on than just looks. And while it's not likely we'll overhaul the world on this concept overnight, I think one of the greatest things we can do to start fighting the constant appearance-based narrative, is to stop contributing to it and focus instead on the things about people that truly matter.

Taking the Focus off Weight

Every magazine you see has headlines touting the next thing that will help you to be 'skinny' or 'slim' or 'thin.' Everything is about losing a certain number of pounds or sizes, or how much the cake/brownie/milkshake we had last night is going to affect our weight.

It's become customary to step on the scale every morning. The number tells us if we've been good or bad the previous day, or over the course of the week. We let that number make or break our whole day! If we see a number that's higher than we expect, how do we tend to react? We restrict. We diet. We don't allow ourselves to have certain foods or drinks. They're now off limits because we 'don't deserve them' because we're already too heavy.

The opposite happens too: we step on, see a lower number than we expected, do a little happy dance, and then permit ourselves to eat more than we otherwise would have as a reward for being so 'good.' We directly tie our eating behavior to what we see on the scale. That darn scale is holding us captive, dictating our every move and causing us to feel bad about ourselves. So it's time we separated our weight and our body from our food.

Yes, it's been drilled into us our whole lives that eating less and moving more means we'll lose weight. And studies have shown over and over again that lowering our calories (either by diet, exercise, or both) means we lose weight. However, that truth doesn't mean we *should* be attaching our food to our weight.

As we've already covered, wanting to lose weight comes from being dissatisfied with the body we have now. I told you that I do not think you should be dissatisfied with your current body. No matter what state it's in, it's the one you have, and it is lovable and awesome just as it is!

However, I also understand the feeling of not being comfortable in your own skin. If you were previously a smaller size or weight than you are now, it can be frustrating to feel so different than you used to feel. Perhaps you had more energy back then or felt happier back then, or perhaps you had fewer aches and pains then, etc. I am not saying that those things don't matter. On the contrary, those are the things that matter! Not your weight!

If Not Weight, What *Do* We Focus On?

Having more energy, feeling happy, being in less pain —those are things we can work on improving, instead of working on losing weight. Weight and size are just a byproduct of behaviors and actions (and a bit of genetics too). Therefore, rather than focusing on *weight*, our focus is better placed on our *actions* and *behaviors*.

I'll harp on the media again for a moment. They are constantly drilling into us that losing weight or dress sizes is the "be-all and end-all" of health. That isn't so. There are heavy people who are healthy, and slim people who are unhealthy. Your weight is not the sole determinant of health.

Instead, your behaviors dictate your health. If we want to bring this back around to nutrition and eating, there are so many reasons to eat healthily and move more that have nothing to do with weight.

If you want to have more energy and fewer aches and pains, move more! Sure, that might end up also producing weight loss, or it might not, but by moving more, you reap so many more benefits than just whatever happens to your weight. You improve your cardiac health (your heart gets more resilient) and respiratory health (you breathe better). You become stronger, and better able to go through life doing any number of feats you want to do – move furniture, play with kids or grandkids, take a hike at a moment's notice, go swimming in the ocean, ride a bike, walk your dogs without getting winded, etc.

The same goes for food. Eating an amount that doesn't leave you feeling stuffed, bloated, and uncomfortable feels good. Eating foods that nourish you and satisfy you feels good, regardless of its effect on your weight.

Getting lots of vitamins and minerals from fruits and veggies can mean that we're covering our nutritional bases so that we have energy, feel vibrant, and experience less malaise. It means getting in antioxidants that help us fight cancer. It means ensuring that we're not deficient in various nutrients. It means we're giving our bodies what they need to maintain our best health.

These are all reasons to eat well that have nothing to do with our weight. Basically, by eating nutritious foods and moving our bodies, we improve our chances of staying on this planet longer and enjoying more years with the people we love. I can't think of a better reason than that!

Being able to enjoy all foods without guilt also means much less stress and anxiety. Of course, brownies aren't ever going to be considered the most nutritious food on the planet. But if you're able to enjoy one and move on with your day, it's much more enjoyable (and way less stressful) than sneaking a whole tray of them in secret because you think they're bad.

There is such freedom that comes from detaching our food from out weight. Yes, attach it to your *health*, certainly. But that includes your mental health (and sanity) just as much as it does your physical health. And your health isn't dependent on your weight; it's dependent on your *behaviors*.

Focus on What You Want in Life

I like to think of it this way: I could be super-model thin, but always hungry, always thinking about food, feeling out of control around sweets because I think I can't eat them, and generally miserable and unhappy. Or I could be just a regular average person, loving life, happy as a clam, and existing in whatever body my happy and healthy choices leave me with.

I pick option #2. I'd rather be happy. And if you're in the same boat, then I encourage you to focus on those things you want out of life; namely, that happiness piece. Happiness is not tied to your weight or your size. You can choose to be happy now, in this body.

Want to know a cool perk of working on the happiness piece first? Being happy and accepting of and loving ourselves means we *want* to take better care of ourselves. We realize that we are worthy of being treated well. That means taking time for self-care, eating in a way that's satisfying and nourishing, not punishing ourselves for anything related to food, and moving in a way that feels good to us.

When we care about someone, we take care of them. And that goes for ourselves too. We can't hate ourselves into a smaller version of us. We'll just be a smaller and more miserable self! Work on the happiness piece. Work on the self-care piece. And you'll notice you *want* to treat yourself well as a result, not as a punishment for having eaten a brownie yesterday.

CHAPTER 6: ACCEPTANCE, SELF-COMPASSION, AND A GROWTH MINDSET

First Step: Acceptance

Before we can start to move away from a place of body dissatisfaction and negativity toward a more positive viewpoint, we first have to accept where we are at this very moment.

We spend a lot of time thinking if we could only lose 10 pounds or 'get rid of the belly,' we'd feel better about ourselves. We put off liking ourselves until some arbitrary goal is achieved or until we start looking like someone who we think is allowed to like how they look.

But we don't have to wait. In fact, waiting does us a huge disservice. By waiting, we reinforce the idea that the person we are now, in this current body, doesn't deserve to like herself. You *do* deserve to like yourself. We all do. No matter what we look like.

The very first step in making headway toward the goal of a better body image is to simply accept where you currently are. You may be a size XXXXXXXXXL, or you may have cellulite, or you may have wrinkles, or you may have a scar the size of Texas across your whole body. It does not matter.

You don't have to like these things if you're not ready for that. At this stage, we're simply working on accepting what currently is true.

I have freckles (even in my eyes), and lots of moles.

I have cellulite.

I have small boobs that still manage to find a way to droop.

I have acne-prone skin.

I have skin that's pale and burns rather than tans.

I have a double chin sometimes.

My butt is flat.

I have scars.

All of these things are true of my body. They may sound like complaints, but they are not. They are just statements of what is true about my body. Any *feeling* about these things is what we'll talk about next, in step two. Step one is simply to accept, without judgment.

Let Go of Things You Can't Change

What's that saying? "Grant me the serenity to accept the things I cannot change"? Many of those things above, I can't change about myself. I can't erase my freckles or un-droop my boobs (at least not without very expensive surgery). I can't change the structure of my chin, my tanning ability, or my cellulite (no matter how many body cream commercials try to convince me otherwise). Some of these things just 'are what they are.' So we free up our brain space considerably if we accept these things we cannot change. Thinking about changing the unchangeable is an exercise in frustration. Accepting and letting go of the things we cannot change becomes a huge burden lifted off our shoulders.

But, what about the things we *could* change? Won't trying to like my body cause me to stop wanting to be healthier or improve anything? In the wonderful words of Carl Roger: "The curious paradox is that when I accept myself just as I am, then I can change."

The answer here lies in the fact that health is about more than just looks or weight. We can accept ourselves as we currently are, and yet still want to make changes. The important thing is that the desire to change comes from a desire for more health and happiness, not wanting to escape your current situation or because you don't like the way you currently look. It's a positive motivation, not a negative one.

For example, someone who is good at a sport doesn't stop practicing. They care enough about their health and happiness to keep practicing and keep improving, even when they're already "good."

The state of our bodies is the same way. We are all already worthy of love, kindness, and respect, just by existing as a human being. It does not matter what the physical shell of a person looks like. From this standpoint, we are all already "good." But we are never a finished product, are we?

We don't call ourselves "good" and then stop doing anything that relates to our health. We still have to eat to continue existing. We still have to move around our world in some way. And if we want to live a long and happy life, it behooves us to take care of the physical shell we inhabit.

In the interest of not waiting until some arbitrary thing is achieved, we can choose to accept our current bodies just as they are and allow ourselves to be happy *now*, even if there are things we still want to improve.

Body Appreciation

When we stop placing so much attention on looks or weight, we are sometimes left to wonder what else we should be focusing on instead. In my opinion, one of the most important things we can redirect our focus to is all the things our bodies can *do*. This is how we build body appreciation.

You have only one body. While it may change in many ways over the course of your life, it is still the only one you have. Appreciate that it allows you to hug your loved ones, play your favorite sport, climb the stairs to your home, and take lovely walks. Your body gives you the ability to do all sorts of wonderful things, and focusing on those can be a big foundational piece of improving our overall body image.

Self-Compassion and Self-Kindness

After acceptance comes compassion. If you're coming from a place of prior self-criticism, then it feels rather fake to suddenly try thinking of ourselves as amazing, or beautiful, or incredible, or fantastic. And that's why I don't recommend trying to make that leap. As much as I would love to tell you I can help you go from disliking your body to believing you're a goddess overnight, I can't do that. And honestly, that's not the actual the goal. The goal is to see ourselves in a more positive light, certainly. And most of us would assume that the path to get there includes boosting our self-esteem. But self-esteem isn't as helpful as self-compassion; and while they may sound like the same thing, they're actually not.

What's Wrong with Self-Esteem?

When we boil it down, self-esteem is boosted by feeling or believing that you're better than others in one way or another. In a constant mental comparison between ourselves and the people around us, seeing ourselves as superior in some way is what boosts our self-esteem and makes us feel good about ourselves.[33]

But this is not what we're after here. Self-esteem makes us feel good, but it keeps us in a trap of constant comparison and wondering how we stack up against everyone else. And the worst part is, it only works when the comparison seems to be in our favor or when we succeed at something.

We feel better and have higher self-esteem when we're the thinnest, or smartest, or whatever-est in the room. But self-esteem completely abandons us when we perceive ourselves as not stacking up, or when we think someone else is better than us in some way. Yet, that's when we most need to feel better![33]

Kristin Neff is one of the lead researchers in this area, and I love how she discusses this idea. I've put some of her quotes below (bolded emphasis is mine):

> **"Self-compassion doesn't demand that we evaluate ourselves positively or that we see ourselves as better than others.** *Rather, the positive emotions of self-compassion kick in exactly when self-esteem falls down; when we don't meet our expectations or fail in some way. This means that the sense of intrinsic self-worth inherent in self-compassion is highly stable. It is constantly available to provide us with care and support in times of need."*[34]

It's not about feeling better than others, as in the case of boosted self-esteem. It's about being kinder to ourselves when we feel less-than. If we're constantly thinking negative things about our bodies, then the goal is to be kinder and more compassionate to ourselves, so we can start to accept where we are and then view things more positively. We're not shooting for thinking we're goddesses; we're shooting for at least *not* thinking negatively about ourselves!

> *"Self-compassion involves being kind to ourselves when life goes awry or we notice something about ourselves we don't like, rather than being cold or harshly self-critical. It recognizes that the human condition is imperfect, so that we feel connected to others when we fail or suffer rather than feeling separate or isolated. It also involves mindfulness — the recognition and non-judgmental acceptance of painful emotions as they arise in the present moment. Rather than suppressing our pain or else making it into an exaggerated personal soap opera, we see ourselves and our situation clearly."*[34]

As you can see, wrapped up in this idea of self-compassion is the idea of acceptance again. Recognizing something and accepting it without judgment helps us avoid being mean to ourselves so we can show ourselves a bit of kindness instead.

How Does This Relate Back to Dieting?

As we've mentioned before, body dissatisfaction is the root cause of dieting and unhealthy weight control behaviors. We can talk about tips and strategies for ditching diets all we want, and they may help for a short time; but that's just treating the symptom. If we can tackle that underlying cause, that is, how we view our bodies, then we erase the urge to diet in the first place!

Trying to ditch dieting before addressing the body image piece is like giving a pain reliever for a broken leg without actually *treating* the break. It might feel better for a while, but the pain will come back until the cause is fixed.

So how do we fix this body image thing? How do we undo the years and years of diet-talk and body negativity? We start first with the acceptance piece above. The acceptance piece then ties in very closely with the compassion piece. Part of self-compassion is kindness, and another part is seeing the bigger picture of common humanity.

We often feel as though we are the only ones feeling this way, like we're the only ones who hate their thighs, while everyone else is off enjoying cellulite-free paradise somewhere. But that's not true. Many more people have cellulite than lack it. And it's very likely that most of those people are also upset by their cellulite. Basically, you're not alone, and realizing that is incredibly helpful!

Self- Kindness Is a Big Part of Self-Compassion

The kindness part of the self-compassion piece is the crucial piece. However, it is sometimes easier to do when we turn the tables around. Instead of thinking about ourselves and how we can show *ourselves* kindness, it can be easier to think of our friends or loved ones, and how we show kindness to *them*.

Imagine if your best friend, or sister, or daughter, thought the same negative things about their bodies that you think about yours. It hurts your heart a bit to think of that, doesn't it? We don't want the people we care about to dislike themselves, because *we* see how awesome they are. The not-so-secret secret here is: They feel the same way about you!

So pretend for a moment that you and your reflection in the mirror are two separate people. Now imagine that reflection is someone you love and care about (your daughter, sister, best friend, etc.). That person now says something negative about her body. How would you respond? I'm willing to bet you wouldn't tell her "Yeah, you're right. Those thighs of yours are totally hideous. You should really do something about that." No, you're kinder than that!

The thing is, we say that mean and negative stuff to ourselves all the time. We look in the mirror, think the person staring back at us is too heavy, or too wide, or too cellulite-y, or too tired-looking, and we belittle that person. We say and think all sorts of mean things about how 'if I could just lose this extra weight, I'd be so much better off' and it's not true.

So what would you honestly say to someone you loved who said similar negative things about herself? Your response would be a bit more compassionate and kind, wouldn't it? Let's take ourselves through this whole process as an example.

Current Diet Mindset Version

We look in the mirror and see all that is 'wrong' with ourselves. We touch our thighs or belly and wish they would get smaller. We feel sad and upset that our body is not looking anything like a cover model, and we interpret that to think that our current body isn't good enough or is unattractive. We tell ourselves how we need to step up our game and go hard-core into dieting and working out again. This time it'll work. This time we'll finally lose the weight and shrink our trouble spots so we can be happy.

Acceptance and Compassion Version

We look in the mirror and see a whole person, one who is not perfect (because none of us are), but who has so many awesome qualities. We see that our thighs or belly may be large, or squishy, and we accept that this is what this body currently looks like. No big deal. We don't get upset about it; instead, we know that we are loved no matter what our body looks like. Since we are already content with ourselves, we think about how we can treat ourselves even *better*, and care for ourselves even more, by doing something that fosters our long-term health.

Do you see the difference? In the first scenario, we're looking at ourselves compared to an unrealistic ideal and trying to force ourselves to change in order to escape the current reality. In the second scenario, we know the person in the mirror is a wholly wonderful human being just as they are, and we only wonder how we can treat them *more* kindly or in a way that fosters their health and happiness.

No human being on this earth is perfect. There is no such thing as a perfect human! We just are who we are, and our bodies are just the physical container. Our love for others and our kindness and respect for others doesn't tend to hinge on whether or not they have cellulite or weigh 600 pounds.

See the person inside. Be kind to the person inside. Have compassion for where that person is in her life and her journey. And please remember: you are not alone.

Self-Kindness Is Not Self-Indulgence

I want to point out one key thing about self-kindness so that we don't confuse it with something else. In thinking back to the question about not wanting to change or improve if we start accepting ourselves, a related question starts to come to mind in terms of self-kindness: If I'm being kind to myself, doesn't that mean I can just do whatever I want that seems nice? Our researcher friend Kristin Neff has a response to this idea in these two amazing quotes [emphasis mine]:

"Our recent findings show that self-kindness can take many forms, and some people described acts of self-kindness to be watching television, indulge and over-indulge on their favorite foods, use recreational drugs, and binge drink. Others said that to be kind to themselves they might take a warm bath, go for a walk, jog, or eat a healthy and nourishing meal. **The former group of behaviors may have negative health consequences (e.g., lead to obesity, cardiovascular disease), while the latter group of behaviors depicts an alignment of self-kindness and self-care, which is perhaps a truer model of self-compassion,** *and has been briefly mentioned in past literature (Neff, 2009, 2011), and relates to the body and mind simultaneously."*[35]

"Many people say they are reluctant to be self-compassionate because they're afraid they would let themselves get away with anything. " I'm stressed out today so to be kind to myself I'll just watch TV all day and eat a quart of ice cream." This, however, is self-indulgence rather than self-compassion. **Remember that being compassionate to oneself means that you want to be happy and healthy in the long term.** *In many cases, just giving oneself pleasure may harm well-being (such as taking drugs, over-eating, being a couch potato), while giving yourself health and lasting happiness often involves a certain amount of displeasure."*[36]

To sum up those two quotes as concisely as possible: Being kind to ourselves means seeking a balance between the short-term and long-term wants, and keeping that long-term desire for health and happiness on our radar.

There may be times when keeping that long-distance view in mind is difficult or challenging, and I believe that's what she meant by "displeasure." Sometimes, like in her example, we want to just watch TV and eat a quart of ice cream to feel better in the moment.

Choosing to find a non-food way of giving ourselves happiness, and also promoting our health in the process, feels difficult at first. But acting in true self-kindness and self-compassion means giving that long-term viewpoint the upper hand when the short-term view doesn't promote our health and happiness.

Develop a Growth Mindset

On the heels of acceptance and self-compassion is the development of something called a Growth Mindset. A growth mindset is the vital next piece of this body image makeover idea. But do you know what that means?

A growth mindset means that you don't view things as set in stone. There is always room for learning, for growth, for improvement. You are not "stuck" in your current state. A growth mindset is the opposite of a fixed mindset, which is essentially settling for the status quo. "It is what it is" and this is how it always will be.

I mentioned before that it's okay to accept things as they are while still wanting to change them. This is where the growth mindset versus a fixed mindset comes in. Wanting to change something, but thinking we're stuck a certain way (a fixed mindset), is upsetting. Wanting to change something and *seeing a way to do that*, on the other hand, is empowering!

Common Fixed Mindsets

Let's first discuss some common fixed mindsets that can develop when we get wrapped up in a diet mindset:

- I'm an emotional eater.

- I can't control myself around cake.

- I'll always be heavy/fat/big – I can't lose weight.

- I'm terrible at cooking.

- Eating healthy is hard.

All of these things may have a glimmer of truth to them. Perhaps you really do tend to turn to food when you're emotional or have a tough time saying no to cake. Perhaps you really have been big/fat/heavy your entire life and have dieted and dieted and haven't lost weight. Maybe your cooking skills aren't very good, and you have a difficult time eating healthily.

It's *okay* to accept these things as they currently are. The key here, though, is not to let the current state become the *only* one your brain sees as possible. That's a fixed mindset. Thinking "Well, that's just how I am" is self-defeating. It leaves no room for learning, or growth, or change. Identifying yourself as an emotional eater means surrendering to the idea that food will always be the only way in which you cope with tough emotions. But we can challenge that narrative.

Growth Mindset Rephrasing

If we rephrase the above statements into growth-mindset statements, we suddenly feel a sense of hope, a sense that we're not actually as stuck as we thought we were:

- I've always eaten in response to tough emotions, *but I can practice trying other ways to deal with them.*

- I really like sweet foods, *but they don't hold power over me*. I can practice finding a moderate approach to them.

- I may be heavy, *but I can make a few changes to my habits or lifestyle to become healthier* and maybe also lose weight along the way.

- I can't cook well *yet*, but I can *learn to make some new things* and practice some cooking skills.

- I'm not a fan of most vegetables, *but I can try new ones* or cook some of them differently to find ones I do like.

In all of these rephrases, the facts haven't changed. Someone who isn't good at cooking doesn't start thinking "I'm a good cook." They're still not good at cooking (yet). So they acknowledge where they currently are, and see that there is a way to improve with practice in the future.

Things that are difficult now get easier with practice. Something you're not good at yet is something you can learn how to do. Having always been one way about something doesn't mean you can't be another way.

The common theme here is that you are not stuck. There is almost always a way forward through something you want to improve. Human beings are capable of great learning, and we are capable of practicing things. Don't assume to be stuck, find a way forward! And as was also mentioned before, come at this idea of changing from a view of wanting more goodness in your life, rather than trying to move away from something negative.

CHAPTER 7: PROMOTING POSITIVE BODY IMAGE IN KIDS

It's Never Too Early to Avoid Weight Comments

If you think back, far back to when you first started to think negatively about your body, you may notice that there were comments from others that planted that seed of negativity in you. When it comes to instilling a positive body image in our kids, our primary objective is to not be the source of those negative comments!

When our kids are very little, we are the main people they look to for pretty much everything. In those formative, early years, there is no need to bring up weight or shape at all, except for a doctor's appointment when they actually get weighed.

It is common, when kids are very little, for people to comment on their bodies. Since we tend to find kids cute and adorable, we think that talking about their "chubby legs" and "big belly" is okay. They are very unlikely to understand this type of talk when they are only a couple of months old, but it is still wise to nip this kind of talk in the bud whenever possible.

There is no need to comment on a child's body or weight, especially if commenting on fatness, chubbiness, or skinniness. Yes I know, in the spirit of acceptance, these things are simply observations (baby legs usually are chubby!). And while there may not be a negative connotation to that phrasing when the comment is made, eventually kids start to pick up on society's negative attitude toward those things. If they've been called chubby their whole lives, and start to realize that chubby is seen as negative to most of society, it can be really upsetting.

If you truly feel the need to comment on their admittedly rapidly changing bodies, keep it to how much they're growing *up* and becoming more capable of awesome things. Leave any talk of body shape or gaining/losing weight out of it, if possible.

Encourage the other adults your child spends a lot of time with to do the same. When kids are so little, it is mostly family and close caregivers who will have the biggest influence. Be sure these people know not to comment on body size, shape, or weight.

Fighting Outside Influences

Eventually, our little birds fly the nest, even if it's only for a short time to go to school and come right home. This is where, unfortunately, they will be subjected to the weight stigma and bullying that is all too common.

We can't prevent other kids from making comments about weight or bullying our kids. As parents, we can simply do our best to mitigate that negativity and fight it by instilling body positivity in our kids. How do we do that? We do it by focusing on body appreciation and modeling/teaching healthy behaviors.

1 – Teach Body Appreciation

"The definition of body appreciation, according to Tracy Tylka, is 'holding favorable opinions toward the body regardless of its appearance, accepting the body along with its deviations from societal beauty ideals, respecting the body by attending to its needs and engaging in healthy behaviors, and protecting the body by rejecting unrealistic media appearance ideals.'"[37] That is a pretty stellar definition!

Our goal when it comes to instilling body appreciation in our kids is to basically give them a shield against the negativity all around them. We talked a lot in a previous chapter about society's ideals and how it contributes to our negative thoughts about our bodies. Those things, unfortunately, aren't going away anytime soon, so we do our best to build our kids up so those things can't get to them.

First, teach kids to love and appreciate their bodies, unconditionally. Bodies evolve and change throughout our lives, and no matter what their body looks like at any given time, it is always worthy of love, appreciation, care, and respect.

This is true regardless of what percentile they're at on their growth charts. Some kids are naturally at the 98th percentile. Others are in the 10th percentile. As long as they're tracking along the same curve, then they are just doing their job of growing up in the body they have.

2 - Don't Comment on Weight or Size

Focus instead on all the awesome things their body can *do*. They can run, jump, tumble, and dance. They can play a sport (if old enough), or enjoy playing and climbing on playgrounds. Our bodies can do so many incredible things, and the more we focus on all those positives, the better we can shrug off negatives from external sources.

"Research also suggests that perceived body acceptance by others is important in how children come to view their bodies. So the family culture around weight and whether a child feels accepted is a key part of the puzzle."[37]

If we are accepting of their bodies, not making comments about weight, shape, or size, and showing them our own love and appreciation all the time, then that alone serves to instill a sense of acceptance and appreciation in themselves. It is like another layer of protection against the comments that they may eventually hear from others.

Think about how comments from others are more easily brushed off when you feel confident about something. If you know that you gave an incredible presentation at work, and your boss and most coworkers also think it was well done, then it's easy to brush off the one person who decides to say it was boring or stupid. If you're not confident in your presentation, though, and you don't have the support of your boss and other peers, that comment will be much more difficult to hear and deal with.

The comment is the same, but the outcome of how it affects you is different, all because of your own confidence, and your perceived acceptance from others who are important to you. Building up our kids' body appreciation and acceptance works the same way!

One more way we can build up that shield of theirs when they get older is to help them take notice, as we have, of the unrealistic weight and beauty standards put out to us by the media and advertising industries. Help them notice the ways body image is preyed upon in advertising, and how models are photo-shopped to "perfection" in posters and magazines. Keeping them aware of the unrealistic ideals that are all around us can help them to be unaffected by them.

3 – Encourage Healthy Behaviors

Part of caring for their body is treating it well. That includes healthy behaviors like eating well and moving. Help to guide them in eating healthy foods and having a positive relationship with it.

Don't restrict foods, and don't glorify healthy foods. Provide structure for meals and snacks. Provide a variety of foods so they can explore new ones and enjoy their favorites too. Find enjoyable ways to get in movement as a family. Kids don't need workouts; they just need to move around and play. Go to a park or playground, play tag, dance to fun music in your living room, go for walks outside, etc. When they get older, let them enroll in activities/sports they enjoy.

None of these things are done to manipulate their bodyweight or their size. These are simply health-promoting behaviors so that their bodies can be healthy and strong, regardless of what that looks like on them.

SECTION 3: GOOD FOODS VERSUS BAD FOODS

CHAPTER 8: HOW A GOOD/BAD FOOD VIEW HARMS US

Let me ask a few questions to start this chapter:

- Have you ever felt guilty about something you ate?
- Have you ever waited until you were alone to eat a certain food in secret?
- Have you ever put a food you weren't allergic to completely off-limits for yourself?
- Have you ever avoided an entire food group?
- Have you ever made a purchasing decision based on the item's low fat, low carb, sugar free, or other healthy label?

If so, you are not alone. These things are amazingly common, and I think almost everyone I know has experienced at least one of the above. Do you know what links them all together?

All of these things stem from a core belief that certain foods are "good" and others are "bad." In this section, we'll go over where that idea comes from, and the big reasons why this view of food isn't helping us.

Why Do We Believe in "Good" and "Bad" Foods?

Short answer: because this idea is everywhere! Every diet under the sun has some version of a good/bad food mentality. There are foods you're allowed to eat while on the diet, and ones you're not. Some foods are deemed healthy, while others are off limits or cheat foods.

And the actual diets are just the beginning. We also get this idea drilled into us in every health-related post you see in the news and on social media. Headlines are either talking about the latest superfood, or about how horrible some other food is for you. Everything is about how healthy or unhealthy something is, whether it is a good food or a bad one. This notion is not doing us any favors.

Remember that Unicorn Frappuccino that was popular everywhere recently? People fell into two camps: either they thought it was cool and wanted to try it, or they were telling you that indulging in something so laden with sugar and artificial ingredients was a very bad decision. How many posts did you see about the "sugar bomb" that it contained or the artificial colors or flavors inside? Posts such as: "People are excited about the Unicorn Frap, but I'm over here on my high horse thinking you are all really bad at self-control." Can we please just stop with the health judgment?

Yes, there are some foods that are healthier than others – they have more nutrients, they're whole or less processed, etc.– but that does not mean they are good.

And foods that are less nutritious, the ones that are very processed, or mostly sugar, or high in fat, or calories, or artificial anything? They are not bad. Nor are we bad people for eating/drinking them. These foods usually taste pretty good actually, so we *want* to eat them. But everything around us is telling us they're bad, and by default, *we* must be bad for allowing ourselves to be tempted by these foods. We are told we are weak, or we lack self-control, or we're "addicted." And we start to believe and internalize this point of view.

This is where we start to see how viewing things in black and white terms of good versus bad is harmful to our relationship with food.

Three Reasons This Thinking Is Harmful

There are three main reasons why viewing foods as either good or bad ruins our relationship with food.

1 – Thinking a food is bad doesn't mean we eat less of it

2 – Restriction feeds binges

3 – This black-and-white viewpoint causes guilt

Reason #1: Telling Us Something Is Bad Doesn't Make Us Want It Less

When you tell your kid not to do something, does that thing then become the only thing they do want to do? There is something very tempting about things we're not allowed to do, or that someone has told us to avoid. It ups the intrigue factor. Things that are bad or off limits become the things that are more interesting! (Anyone who ever had a crush on one of the "bad boys" back in high school knows what I'm talking about!)

Having such a black-and-white (otherwise known as "dichotomous") view of foods is common among dieters. What's interesting is that people who have a very rigid approach to dietary restraint (view foods as good or bad, and themselves as being on or off diets) are more likely to gain weight back than people who follow a more flexible approach.[38] In fact, in one study that specifically looked at psychological factors preceding weight regain, "the most powerful predictor of weight regain was dichotomous thinking."[39] This may be partly due to more intense or frequent food cravings when someone takes a more rigid, black-and-white approach. "[R]igid eating behaviors lead to food cravings, thereby hampering long-term weight maintenance. Indeed, people with flexible control strategies have been found to be more successful in long-term weight maintenance."[40]

Additionally, if people move from a rigid dietary viewpoint to one that is more flexible, they have an easier time managing or maintaining their weight, their psychological distress *decreases*, and their general well-being improves![41]

Essentially, the rigid mindset of seeing foods as only either good or bad makes eating more stressful. When we view things more flexibly, our psychological well-being improves.

Calling a food "bad" doesn't mean you'll eat less of it. It means that the food becomes even more tempting; and since it's so tempting, we try even harder to put it off limits. It becomes another cycle, where we see a food as bad, become more tempted by it, and then see it as even worse because now it's not just "bad," it's also something we're drawn to. Eventually, this cycle can get the better of us, and we end up eating that off-limits food ... and it's hard to stop once we start. This is where reason #2 comes in ...

Reason #2: Restriction Feeds Binges

We've discussed body dissatisfaction and how that leads to dieting, and we just covered how viewing foods as good or bad causes us to want those "bad" foods even more. Now, we're talking about how the combination of those two things can lead to a behavior many of us have engaged in but wish we could stop: bingeing.

I know, bingeing is associated with actual eating disorders (which are *not* part of this book). But even well before the development of a full-blown eating disorder, there is a basic truth that exists: restriction feeds binges.[40]

Putting delicious things completely off limits because we consider them to be bad only serves to make them more enticing. And while we can usually 'white-knuckle it' through the restriction for a while, there often comes a point when it becomes too difficult. Eventually, it starts to make us feel so bad, we decide to say, "Forget this!" That's when binges happen.

We have probably all experienced the semi-out-of-control feeling when we finally let in some super delicious food we'd been avoiding for a while. We finally get a taste of the 'forbidden fruit' and we say, "Wow, this is so good, I can't stop!" We feel like something outside of ourselves takes over and it's like autopilot to just keep finding more and more delicious food or sweets to fill our mouths and bellies with. In the back of our minds we still view it as bad, so we figure we might as well get as much of it in as we can now, because it'll be off-limits again once we stop.

The root cause of that binge behavior is restriction. And why do we restrict things? We restrict them because we think they're bad, which leads me to the final reason this dichotomous thinking is harmful ...

Reason #3: A Black-and-White Viewpoint Causes *Guilt*

What happens when we do find ourselves bingeing and finally stop? We usually feel guilty about having so much of those "bad" foods, right? It goes back to what I mentioned in the first chapter: diets cause us to feel guilty, and that guilt causes us to make more decisions we don't like.

Here's how the good/bad point of view fits into the whole diet/guilt cycle:

- Seeing a food as bad makes it even more appealing.
- The added appeal makes it very difficult *not* to eat the food.
- When we do eventually give in and eat it, and we remember just how delicious it is, we can't stop at a reasonable amount.
- We then feel guilty for eating the food in the first place, and for eating so much of it.
- We feel bad about ourselves, about our resolve, and about our ability to eat well.
- Then we usually figure "Well, I already messed up, I might as well make it worth it," and we end up eating even *more* foods

that we've deemed bad, which just keeps the cycle of shame and indulgence going.

- Since we feel so bad, we shun the "bad" food even more, restricting it more than before, and causing the cycle to start again.

Do you remember where guilt comes from? It comes from betraying our values or standards. When we view foods as bad, and then we eat those foods (or a lot of those foods), we feel like we betrayed our value of eating healthfully. We view those foods as completely outside of something a "healthy" person would eat, and so we view our actions as something to be deeply ashamed of.

What If We Simply Viewed Food As Food, Instead?

What if we took the "bad" judgment off them? We wouldn't feel as though we betrayed anything! We'd think, "That was a super yummy brownie" and move on with our lives. We can be a healthy person who occasionally eats brownies. No one magically becomes an unhealthy person by eating a brownie.

Our overall eating pattern encompasses a huge amount of food if we look at it over the course of a week, or a month, or a year. If you eat *mostly* brownies, then yes, you probably won't feel your best. But if the majority of your eating is healthy and wholesome , then the few less-healthy foods sprinkled in here and there honestly don't matter much at all.

Taking a more middle-of-the-road approach and allowing all those things we used to put off limits diminishes their power tremendously. Those foods no longer control us, we regain *our* power and control, and the foods become no big deal anymore – it's all just food! The key is to stop restricting so rigidly. And believe me, I know that sounds terrifying. But after a short adjustment, we realize "Wow, this is what freedom feels like!"

Ditch the Healthy Eating Perfectionism

There is no such thing as perfect when it comes to eating. No one on this planet eats "perfectly." When we're working on eating a bit healthier, it's easy to slip into perfectionism, thinking everything we eat needs to be good for us, and we fail if we eat something bad. Chasing perfection, especially when it comes to food, is just an exercise in frustration. Nothing will ever be good enough when we're striving for perfection or categorizing foods into good versus bad.

To stop thinking in black and white, we have to embrace the grey. Grey is neutral, even though it still has various shades. What I mean by that is: Yes, some foods are healthier than others. But there is no moral judgment here. All foods are just foods, even though they are different foods. Instead of dividing foods into good and bad buckets, take a more neutral approach and put all foods on one level, with nothing on a pedestal and nothing shunned forever.

I get it; grey is boring. But you know what? This little analogy totally works with colors too. There are no bad colors, just different shades and hues that make up the bigger category of color, even though they're all different. And food is the same. There is no moral attachment to any of them. It's all just food.

When you first hear the suggestion to view all foods neutrally, it's normal to be taken aback. It doesn't seem to make sense at first, does it? Viewing foods as totally neutral sounds lovely, but there *are* differences between foods. If we want to eat healthily, then surely we can't just eat brownies all day, even though they're yummy and still "just food," right?

And that is true. But the key difference here is that we start to move away from labeling something as "bad" and, instead, view it as just a piece of an overall bigger picture. It is possible to eat in an overall healthy manner, one that includes some less-nutritious foods sometimes, and not deem the less-healthy foods to be "bad." How do we do that? By using an approach I call the Two-Spectrum Approach, which is the focus of the next chapter.

CHAPTER 9: A BETTER VIEW: THE TWO-SPECTRUM APPROACH TO FOOD

I know it's easy to assume that I've always approached food in the neutral way that I do now, but that's not actually true. Like many people, I came from a background of viewing certain foods as good or bad. Going back to school for my Nutrition degree actually reinforced this. Anything that wasn't super healthy was either ignored or talked about only in terms of how it would most certainly cause a decline in health.

Plus, as someone wanting to help others to eat well, I figured my own eating had to be picture perfect. I had to set a good example, right? I'd be at a restaurant and feel like I shouldn't order the thing I wanted, because a healthy person would just order a salad. Or I'd think that I couldn't have cake at a party because I'm "the healthy one" and healthy people aren't supposed to eat cake.

I will tell you right now, that is a total lie. Healthy people *can* eat cake. And they *can* order things they enjoy off the dinner menu. Remember that there is no such thing as perfection in eating!

So how did I eventually come to see food in a more neutral light? I started to shift my mindset. I went from thinking things like "brownies are *bad* and I should avoid them" to "I love brownies and I just want to make sure to eat them in moderation."

Oh No, There's That "Moderation" Word!

"Everything in moderation" is something people have such a love/hate relationship with. But if we're embracing the idea that foods aren't good or bad, and we're not seeking perfectionism in eating, then "everything in moderation" ends up being a pretty great way of concisely describing this overall approach.

- It's inclusive of all foods.
- It's not shaming of any particular food or food group.
- It covers the general idea that just about anything can fit into an overall healthy eating lifestyle, as long as we don't go overboard.

All foods are just foods. Anything can fit. Everything is on the table, and we are free to choose from a plethora of options. However, we know that eating only one food group for the rest of our lives wouldn't be a healthy choice. So rather than eat only brownies, or only carbs, or only fat, since those are enjoyable things and they're allowed and not "bad" anymore, we just include them *among* the other foods that make up an overall healthy eating pattern.

So how do we put this "everything-in-moderation" approach together with the desire to eat in a way that still promotes our overall health? My answer to that question is something I call the Two-Spectrum Approach. Let's take a look at the two spectrums I'm talking about:

Spectrum #1: A Way to Look at Individual Foods

The first spectrum is the one on which a single food rests. It goes from "Less nutritious" to "More nutritious."

Spectrum #1: Where individual foods lie

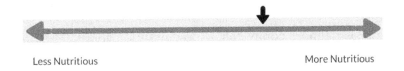

Less Nutritious   More Nutritious

Foods themselves are not good or bad, but they *do* differ in their nutritional impact. Some foods are full of healthy vitamins, minerals, antioxidants, fiber, and other health-promoting components. Others have very little of that nutritious stuff in addition to their calories (but they tend to taste really good!).

Every single food falls somewhere on the spectrum between more nutritious and less nutritious. Vegetables, fruits, lean proteins, whole grains, and heart-healthy fats all contain more health-promoting components than brownies, for example.

That doesn't make those things "good" and brownies "bad," though. These things simply differ in their nutritional content. That's a fact. Facts are still facts; it's the *judgment* of those facts that we want to avoid. Because thinking a food is "bad" only serves to instill a sense of guilt about enjoying it. And we've already covered how guilt isn't helpful.

Spectrum #2: A Way to View Our Overall Eating Pattern

The second spectrum is where our overall eating pattern falls. If we were to look at every food we ate over the course of a week or a month, we'd see that the total of all those things falls somewhere on this spectrum.

The scale here is the same: "Less nutritious" to "More nutritious." The less nutritious side would be an eating pattern composed almost completely of low-nutrition foods. The other end would be composed almost completely of whole, unprocessed, kissed-by-a-unicorn, nutrition-for-the-sole-purpose-of-fueling-your-body-no-matter-what-it-tastes-like foods.

Spectrum #2: Where our overall eating pattern lies

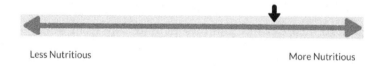

Less Nutritious   More Nutritious

If you're, you know, *human*, you fall somewhere in the middle. What's cool about thinking about it this way, is that we start to realize that each food has a very small impact on the bigger picture. No single food moves us up or down this second spectrum all that much! If your eating consists of mostly whole foods, throwing in a brownie or a slice of cheesecake here and there doesn't suddenly shift you from the healthier side of the spectrum to the less healthy side. It would take eating *mostly* brownies and cheesecake to shift your eating pattern that far on the spectrum. This is really encouraging! It takes the focus off the minuscule details of one individual food and allows us to see how it fits within a bigger picture view.

So all foods can fit. *How much* of a particular food you want to include will determine how it affects your overall eating spectrum. My mentor Georgie Fear has said, "There is a weight-loss portion of every food," and while this book is not about losing weight, I think the sentiment is still applicable. We don't need to be afraid of foods or put anything off limits, ever. Just because a particular food is more fun than functional doesn't mean it's bad. It just means we fit it in around all the other awesome nutrition-packed foods.

When looking at this from a perspective of long-term health, all you need to ask yourself is: "Does most of my eating fall on the 'more nutritious' side of the spectrum?" If so, then you're already doing great! And if you find that the majority of your eating is on the "less nutritious" side, but you're concerned about your long-term health, then you can choose to make some changes to try to shift closer to the "more nutritious" side of the spectrum if you want to.

Where on the spectrum you feel best will be a very individual thing. Some people will want to include more "less nutritious" foods than others. And that doesn't make them, or their choices, bad. Again, there is no moral judgment here.

The key takeaway is this: All foods can fit when we take a bigger picture overview of our eating pattern. A healthy eating pattern can absolutely include things like brownies and cheesecake sprinkled among all the other more nutritious foods! (Thank goodness, right?) The bigger overall picture is what matters most.

CHAPTER 10: HOW TO EAT HEALTHILY WITHOUT DIETING

This book is about mindset first and foremost, so the focus is not on telling you *what* to eat. However, I totally understand that if you're doing all this work to unravel a diet mentality, you probably want some guidance on how to eat in a generally healthy way without the diet mindset calling the shots.

Rules are made to be broken, as they say. So you won't get new rules here to replace the old diet mindset ones. Instead, the idea is to find a flexible strategy that works well for you and your family. We'll cover my approach to healthy meals first, then get into detail on how I manage the less-nutritious foods in a sane and flexible way.

A Healthy Meal Template

In talking specifically about meals, the simplest guidance I can give you is this: Shoot for balanced meals as often as possible. By balanced, I mean one that follows this very general template:

- Include a generous portion of veggies and/or fruits
- Include a protein source

- Include a side serving of whole grains or starchy carbs

- Include a source of fat

- Prioritize whole foods

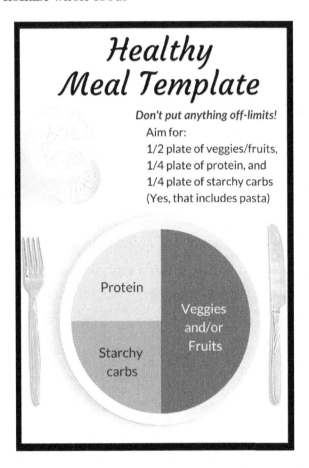

That's it. You'll notice that it's intentionally vague in terms of how much of each thing to include, but that some things are emphasized over others (a "generous" serving of produce versus a "side serving" of starchy carbs, for example). I hope you'll also notice how all the macros are in here: carbs, fat, protein … nothing is demonized, they all get included!

And that's as much guidance as I want to give here because one thing I definitely do not want is for you to take this guidance as a new set of rules to follow. It is simply a suggestion for how to build a healthy meal without dieting.

How much to eat is dependent on your body's signals of hunger and satiety, which we'll cover in the next section. The basic premise is that instead of using some abstract suggested serving size, calorie count, or points tally, you instead use your own internal signals to guide how much to eat.

Use this template when you're meal planning, ordering food, or reheating leftovers. It works in all kinds of situations, which is kind of the point ... it's got to be flexible! And speaking of meal planning, I highly recommend it. Planning your meals in advance helps you save money by only buying what you need, and it helps to eliminate the dreaded "what should we have for dinner" conversation from happening every single night! Not only that, but it helps you plan meals in such a way that you can make sure to include a variety of nutritious foods, as well as some less-nutritious foods you want to enjoy as well!

A Flexible Strategy for Treats

The basic idea for managing less-nutritious foods is to sprinkle them in periodically, without making them a large portion of your overall intake. This applies to things like fried foods, sweets, and alcohol. I tend to speak mostly about sweets, but the concepts can be applied to other less-nutritious foods too.

I also want to point out that some foods that are commonly demonized, like pizza, burgers, etc., may not be overly nutritious, but I find they are more easily incorporated into a meal and balanced out with other more nutritious foods, so I'd approach them using the general meal template described previously. This part is for the sweet stuff and other things people tend to consider "treats" or "extras."

Setting Boundaries

If we want to keep these foods from taking over our intake, we have to set limits or boundaries somewhere. Uh oh, I said "limits." When we start to impose any type of boundary or limitation on food, it can sometimes trigger a bit of an emotional response, or bring up some feelings of restriction that remind you of dieting. But don't fear! We're not getting into dieting territory. There are loads of things in life that we set boundaries on without such an emotional attachment. Some of the best examples are ones we set as parents:

- We let our kids run, but we don't let them run into the street.

- We let our kids play outside, but only where we can see them.

- We let our kids color, but we don't let them color on the walls.

Now think of the common boundaries we set for ourselves:

- We spend money on things we enjoy (like vacations!), but not to the point where can't pay our mortgage.

- We drink alcohol, but we don't drive when we're under the influence (at least I sure hope not!)

- We make plans with friends, but we do so around our other responsibilities and obligations.

In all of these examples, the things in question are all fun and enjoyable things (like coloring or going on vacation), but they have boundaries. There comes a point when the risk/benefit ratio is no longer in our favor.

Enjoying sweets is the same way. They're enjoyable to eat, and we tend to want them every time we see them, just like kids do. When my clients talk about having difficulty managing sweets, you'd be surprised how many describe it as having an impatient inner toddler who just wants the sweet NOW! But if we don't want our kids (or ourselves) to gobble every cookie we see, or eat a candy bar every time we go through the checkout line, then we have to set some boundaries somewhere. Try to view these boundaries unemotionally, just like you view the boundaries listed above. What it comes down to, is that we need the ability to say "no" without it being because the food is "bad."

How to Set Those Boundaries

There are lots of various options you can use to keep the less-nutritious foods within whatever boundaries you're comfortable with. First, decide what a reasonable approach to these foods looks like to you. What *are* your boundaries? Is there a certain upper limit to what you think is reasonable to have in a single day, or maybe within a week? (I should note that in this chapter, I'm mostly talking about your own personal approach to these foods. We'll cover how to handle these boundaries with children in the next chapter, although many aspects are very similar.)

I like to think of things in terms of portion and frequency... as one goes up, the other goes down. For example, if you like large slices of cake, you'd want to enjoy them less frequently. If you prefer something smaller, like a square of chocolate, you could have it more often.

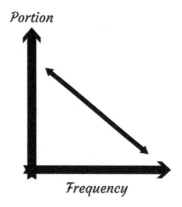

Figure out what works for you and your family. Maryann Jacobsen calls this a "Flexible Goodies Policy" in her book *How to Raise a Mindful Eater*. She does a wonderful job of discussing this if you want to read more. And since I love that terminology, I hope she won't mind me using it in this book as well!

Once you decide on a "policy," it becomes your boundary and your reason for saying "no" to offerings outside the policy. In this way, when we decline a less-nutritious food, it's not because the food is "bad," but because we're simply keeping this type of food at a level that keeps our overall eating pattern one that leans toward being more nutritious.

Remember that your policy should be flexible, though. If it's too rigid, it becomes like diet rules all over again. We want to be able to weigh an unexpected offering against other things we've eaten recently to decide whether or not to eat it.

How It Looks in Practice

The first thing I do when encountering an offer of something yummy but not very nutritious is to figure out if I actually *like* that item. That sounds silly, I know. But if we want to keep the less-nutritious food at a more moderate level, one of the ways to do that is to only choose the ones that we really love and enjoy. We don't need to eat it just because it's there. We want to really enjoy the less nutritious foods that we eat!

So take a moment to think of some things that are your favorites, which you'll almost always want to say "yes" to. Then think of some items that you don't really like all that much. For me, the things I don't enjoy include vanilla cake, candy that isn't chocolate, and dry, store-bought cookies with a ton of frosting. I'll pass on those pretty easily, without feeling deprived. So think of some of the things you can pass on without really missing, and then practice declining those so that the other things you do enjoy can be the ones that get included.

Next, think about the portions and frequency you're comfortable with for some of the things you enjoy. For me, my flexible goodies policy looks like this (specifically about sweets in my case):

- Eat it with, or as part of, a meal whenever possible.
- Aim for either a small amount of something over the course of a few days or a bigger item a couple of times in a week.

That's pretty much it! It's very flexible, and that is on purpose. I know that by having either a little bit each day for a few days, or a bigger thing a couple of times a week, my eating will remain mostly nutritious, and so I don't worry about the details. I don't have a "rule" of eating one piece of chocolate a day, or only eating cake on weekends or having ice cream once per week.

This policy is also very fluid. On the day that I'm writing this, I remember that I went out for ice cream two days ago. It was a larger portion than I'd usually have, and it was also completely separate from a meal. So knowing that I already had one bigger less-nutritious thing recently, I'm not planning on having more large items this week. If something comes up, I'll decide then, but I'm not making a specific plan to go seeking another larger item like a slice of cheesecake. I did buy a lower calorie frozen item to keep in the freezer, though, and I'll have a small amount of it a few times this week when I decide I want to have some after a meal.

There's no beating myself up over the ice cream. There's no restricting or putting anything off-limits to make up for it. There is instead a conscious choice to have smaller servings when I do want a sweet these next few days, and not planning for more instances of bigger sweets.

Your policy may look different, and that's okay! Some people/families like to have one sweet thing per day, usually for dessert after dinner. If another sweet comes up earlier in the day, then there is a choice to be made between that one or having one after dinner.

Other families don't serve dessert each day (including mine). In this case, each dessert opportunity is taken on a case-by-case basis. As you can see in my personal policy, that usually means something small as often as every day, or something bigger less frequently.

Less-nutritious foods that aren't sweets can be treated the same way. Just think of which foods you enjoy that are less nutritious, and devise your strategy for how often you'd ideally like to include them, both for yourself and for how often you serve those things at family meals.

Help Saying "No"

When trying to stick to your policy, eventually you'll come across times where you'll have to say "no" to something if you want to stick to your boundary. There are a few questions I've learned to ask myself that can help:

1 – Do I Actually Really Like This Food Item?

If I don't enjoy it, then it's not worth the extra less-nutritious calories, is it? It's not contributing to my happiness nor to my long-term health, so it's easier to say 'no.'

2 – What Am I Saying 'Yes' to By Saying 'No' to This Food?

Another great concept I learned from Georgie Fear was that every time we say no to something, we are also saying yes to something else. By saying no to this food, we say yes to sticking to our plan. We say yes to keeping our long-term health a priority. We say yes to feeling comfortable (versus overeating, which is so easy to do with sweets, at least for me). We say yes to practicing delayed gratification. There are lots of yes things behind every no, and it can make the "no" easier to say.

3 – When Can I Next Have Something Similar, or That I Enjoy More?

Saying "no" now doesn't mean "no" forever. It is more like a "not right now" than an outright "no." If you know you're going out for ice cream tonight with friends, or you have a date tomorrow to get an indulgent latte, it makes it easier to pass up the cookies a co-worker brings to the office this afternoon. Being able to look forward to an enjoyable food/drink you know you'll have soon helps you move past the immediate disappointment of not getting something right this very moment. (This strategy also works well with kids, as I'll cover in the next chapter!)

These three questions help put an offered temptation into perspective and can be helpful when you're working on staying within your goodies boundaries.

When Adding Forbidden Foods Is Scary

If you're coming from a place where you previously put a lot of foods off-limits, sometimes the idea of reintroducing these things is overwhelming. You feel afraid that allowing these things back in means you'll gorge yourself on them, or not be able to control yourself. Fair warning: that *can* happen. But it's temporary. It's also avoidable if we baby-step into this.

Let's take an example: My client "Mary" had previously considered pizza, burgers, Mexican food, ice cream, brownies, and candy to be "bad" foods, and wouldn't allow herself to eat them. However, when she would go on vacation, she'd allow these foods back in, and then eat *a lot* of them. She is now understandably scared to try allowing these foods back at home since her only experience with allowing them has ended up with her overeating and feeling uncomfortable and upset.

This example shows how restricting something makes it even more enticing. Putting something off-limits completely makes it incredibly hard to keep portions reasonable when you do decide to let those things back in! The key to preventing this is to create a situation that is as easy to handle as possible.

For Mary, this means that once she decides to allow these foods back into her regular eating pattern, she doesn't go 'hog wild' and host a burger, pizza, and ice cream party! Instead, she picks *one* of these foods and chooses ahead of time how she *wants* to incorporate it into an upcoming meal.

Maybe she'll plan to have pizza on Friday night. Or maybe she wants to grill cheeseburgers over the weekend. She doesn't plan on doing both and then following that up with ice cream for dessert. She picks *one* and makes a plan for it.

In keeping with the balanced meal idea mentioned earlier, we also can figure out how these things fit into that flexible meal structure. For the pizza, maybe she orders a slice or two of her favorite topping and a side salad to go with it. For the burgers, she plans to grill some veggies to go alongside the cheeseburger and bun.

In both of these situations, the previously forbidden food is just food. The pizza has carbs, fat, and maybe some protein. So she adds a side salad to get in some veggies and maybe more protein (depending what's on the pizza or in the salad). The cheeseburger on a bun has protein, fat, and carbs, so she rounds it out with veggies to balance the overall meal.

The idea is to make it as easy as possible for you to stick to a portion of the food that you feel good about. If that's two slices of pizza, don't order a whole pie. It can be too tempting to keep going when the rest of the pizza is staring at you.

Create a situation in which you will certainly succeed! Do this a few times, and you'll start to see that you *are* capable of eating these things in a portion that feels good. Once you have the confidence that you can do that, you can try trickier situations (like ordering the whole pizza and taking home leftovers). Think of it like baby steps, and you'll be off and running with your newfound food freedom soon enough!

CHAPTER 11: AVOIDING GOOD/BAD FOOD VIEWS IN KIDS

Like many of the kid-specific chapters in this book, the way in which we convey a mindset of good and bad foods to our kids is through our words and actions. Things we say can impart messages that we may not have intended to send, so it's great to be mindful of the phrases that are, and aren't, helpful.

Things We Say That Convey a Good/Bad Foods Message

"Eat your ___; it's good/healthy for you."

"Don't eat ___, it's bad/unhealthy for you."

"There's too much [fat/sugar/sweetener/food dye/etc.] in that, so don't eat it."

"___ will rot your teeth."

"You need to eat this to grow up big and strong."

Like all things we say to our kids, the intention behind these phrases is a good one. We just want them to eat some nutritious food so they'll grow up healthy. We want their eating to be mostly nutritious food, with just some of the less-nutritious foods sprinkled in (rather than the main focus). And we try to guide them that way by using phrases like these.

But we can still work toward our goal without using terminology that talks about foods being "good" or "bad." The best way we do that is by providing variety and leading by example. We don't need to bribe them to eat the broccoli because it'll make them big and strong. We just provide it with the meal, along with a variety of other foods, and they choose which things to eat from the things that are served.

This way of approaching child feeding is part of Ellyn Satter's Division of Responsibility (DOR), which is brilliant in its simplicity. It says that the parent is responsible only for *what* is served, and *when* and *where* it is served. Children are the ones who are responsible for *whether* or not they will eat, and *how much* they eat.

One of the primary lessons I get out of this DOR style of feeding is that I have to let go of my desire to control how my son eats. We're so used to being totally in control and calling the shots. Or at least, we *think* we're in control. But thinking we're the ones in control is actually what causes some of the frustration. So to lessen the frustration that comes with feeding, we have to let go of some control and be okay with our child choosing not to eat.

Kids are human, and even though they're young and just learning about the world (including the world of eating), they don't need us to control every little thing. They have to take the reins in small steps along the way, and that includes eating. What's so nice about this feeding style is that there is no pressure to eat or not eat things. We just focus on the things we *can* control, the what, when, and where, and let the kids decide to eat or not. Extremely simple in theory. Rather challenging in practice, I admit. But sometimes we have to let go and trust them!

The reason that your child is in charge of whether or not to eat, and how much to eat, is because kids are very well tuned in to their innate hunger and fullness signals. Their little bodies are great at self-regulating their intake, as long as we allow them to do so. You may have noticed this when your kid was an infant and would stop nursing or sucking on the bottle when they were done. You didn't need to coax them to have more; you trusted that their tummy was done (and would be ready for more again later). And even if you did try to coax them to have more, they would turn their head away. When they're done, they're done! The same is still true, even when they're a bit older. They are very good at listening to their hunger and fullness cues!

"But if they don't eat, won't they be hungry later?" Most likely, yes. Just like you would be if you weren't hungry for lunch but got hungry later on. This is totally normal! But I get it. You don't want your kid to refuse his lunch only to ask for a snack 10 minutes later. So, depending on the age of your child, it's helpful to get some expectations put in place.

Three Steps to Implementing The DOR in Your Home

1 -Structure Your Meal/Snack Times

Remember that you are in charge of when and where. This means that you decide when lunch is served, and when snack is served. You do have some flexibility here of course, as you can choose to shift lunch a little earlier or later depending on a particular day's needs and if your child seems to be legitimately hungry or not hungry. But they don't make the final call, you do.

So if it's lunchtime, and they don't want to eat, let them know that it's fine not to eat if they're not hungry. But remind them when the next time they will have a meal or snack will be: "You don't have to eat it if you're not hungry, but we're not having snack until after your nap (or in two hours, or when daddy gets home, etc.)."

If this seems a bit mean, and like you're completely ignoring their actual hunger cues, I hear you. I felt that way at first too. But kids are much more resilient than we give them credit for. And since you're still in charge of when snack is served, you can choose to shift it slightly earlier if you think they're super hungry. They will not starve, I promise. There will be at most 2-3 hours until they can eat again, and if they're not hungry right now anyway, they will very likely be fine to wait.

Having a structure to meal and snack times helps them to eventually regulate their appetite. They'll be able to understand what hunger feels like, and that it's not an emergency that must be fixed as soon as possible. There is always another food opportunity around the corner, and a short while of waiting is healthy and perfectly okay.

(Obviously, keep their age in mind here. If they're 18 months, their tummy is smaller than a 5-year-old and they can't go as long, so you can put your meals and snacks a little closer together.)

A key thing to help with this: Close the kitchen in between feedings. This helps you keep to your structure and prevents kids from grazing, so they can get hungry for meals.

2 - Prevent Picky Eating by Serving Family Style

You are in charge of what is served, but your child still decides whether or not to eat it. To prevent the dreaded "I don't want that" from applying to the entire meal, try serving things in a deconstructed family style way. Think of things like a taco bar, where all the individual pieces are separate and people can take what they want. This idea applies to many more meals than you might first think. Pasta dishes can be served with the pasta, mix-ins, and sauce in separate containers, meat and veggies and potatoes can all be served as separate dishes, etc. The key is to include at least one thing that you know your child likes. This way, there is always something on the table they can eat.

3 - Be Okay with Them Eating Only One Thing

Yes, I fully realize this is the hardest part, and I'm still working on being okay with this myself. If I serve tacos (tortillas, cheese, meat, peppers, and avocado, all separate), and my son only eats tortillas, it's a bit annoying, but I try to allow him to make that choice. If I ask him to eat the other options, it's in a very non-pushy way, like "It might be fun to wrap some peppers in there; want to try?"

Sometimes he will eat only the tortilla and cheese, other times he gobbles the peppers like they're going out of style. And sometimes all he wants is avocado. It sounds strange, but it really does even itself out in the long run. My son usually dislikes chicken, but we still serve it alongside other things he likes. Yesterday he surprised me by not eating things he usually loves (potatoes and eggplant), and eating only the chicken!

Trust them to choose what to eat, and work on letting go of the desire to control it completely. You'll never be able to control it completely anyway, so this saves you (and them) a huge load of frustration and keeps meal times much more pleasant because you're not spending the entire time trying to force them to take one more bite of their broccoli!

Navigate the Less-Nutritious Food by Being in Charge of When, Where, and What

Part of being the role model and guide for our kids in terms of eating is setting those boundaries around the less-nutritious foods. We establish them for ourselves, and also for them. If we don't want them eating cake every day, we don't offer cake every day! Offer sweets within the boundaries you're comfortable with.

But not everything is within our control, and sometimes more opportunities for sweets arise than we'd ideally like. So just like when we help ourselves stay within our boundaries, we have to help them as well. We do that by saying "no" when needed. The key is to give a reason (that is not "because it's bad for you") and to also lessen the disappointment by telling them the next time they'll get something similar.

Here Are Some Examples:

- "I know you want a cookie now, sweetie, but we're having lunch in a little while, and I don't want you to spoil your appetite. We can have dessert after dinner tonight, instead."

- "We already had a cupcake at the party this afternoon, so we're not going to have ice cream after dinner tonight too. Maybe we can go out for ice cream this weekend, though."

- "You really want more candy, but we've had a few pieces already today. We'll put the rest away for now and we can have some more tomorrow."

Notice how there is no mention of the food being "bad." There is just the general message that we don't want to have this type of food as a big piece of our eating pattern.

The Overall Approach

Focus on providing lots of yummy nutritious options in general meals and snacks, and then don't worry too much about including some less-nutritious items into the mix periodically too. Figure out how much works for you and your family, and stick to that. Set your boundaries for your flexible policy on the less-nutritious foods, and then use that to control the when, what, and where of how these foods are offered as best you can.

SECTION 4: HUNGER AND FULLNESS BODY SIGNALS

CHAPTER 12: WE'VE BEEN IGNORING OUR BODY SIGNALS

In my work with clients, we talk a lot about eating according to our hunger and fullness signals. In a perfect world (you know, the kind that doesn't actually exist), we'd eat only using these signals as our guides. But that starts to become kind of like a rule, doesn't it? And we don't like rules. If we're using *guidelines*, though, it does make a lot of sense to use these signals as our guides most of the time.

In this section, we'll talk about ways in which we override or even attempt to manipulate our body signals. Counting calories, clearing our plates, and white-knuckling it through too much hunger are all ways that we put our attention outside of our body's natural cues.

Calorie/Macro/Points Counting

We all know that calories matter if we're trying to lose weight. When we diet or try to lose weight, the idea is to take in less calories than we expend through our activity. When we're trying to maintain our weight, or avoid gaining it, we have to take in the same amount that we burn. This isn't news to you, I know.

Every diet has its own way of getting you into some level of calorie deficit. Some give you pre-portioned shakes or special foods so you don't have to measure or count anything. Others convince you that if you're going to eat food out in the real world, without it being pre-portioned, that you must count the calories (or macros or points) in your food in order to be successful. Diets have convinced us that micro-managing our food is the answer. Doesn't that sound like a fun way to live for the rest of your life? (I hope the sarcasm in those words comes through!)

We don't need to weigh, measure, count, and track every last calorie to make sure that we take in an appropriate amount. Sure, you could do that, if you really and truly wanted to. But if we're interested in peace and happiness in addition to our health, then really, why would you want to do it?

In addition to being a total pain to actually do that, it's also something I'm willing to bet most of us wouldn't want our children to copy from us. That's a barometer by which I try to evaluate my own actions… would I want my son to do this? Our kids learn from everything we do. They're watching. And if we want to raise happy and healthy eaters, we don't want to model food micro-management if we can help it.

There are two underlying reasons that I think we want so much to control our eating:

1. We believe that we can't be trusted. Or rather, we believe that we can't trust our bodies to give us reliable signals to guide our eating in a way that won't end with us gaining a ton of weight.

2. Leaving it up to body signals feels like leaving it to chance, and we prefer to be more organized than that.

I get it. I totally get it. I consider myself to be a bit of a control freak about certain things. I am a planner by nature, and it feels good to me to feel like I have a plan in place to follow. It helps me to feel like I'm organized and that life isn't quite so chaotic. But we can have organized guidelines to follow without giving ourselves strict rules and calorie budgets.

Let's talk about the bigger, more concerning piece though… the *trust* piece. Somewhere along the way, diets convinced us that we can't trust ourselves. They told you that not counting was what got you to the point of wanting to diet. So obviously, if you leave yourself to your own devices, you'll just eat and eat and eat and keep getting fatter and fatter. So they seem to say.

The truth is calorie counts are notoriously unreliable. Measuring our calorie expenditure is also notoriously unreliable. Even when the numbers work out and we see success in terms of pounds lost on the scale, we end up having all the numbers playing mind games with us. So why drive ourselves crazy meticulously counting everything if it's all a big guess and it also drives us bonkers?

How It Interferes with Our Hunger and Fullness Cues

I counted calories for a long time in what now feels like a previous life. I'm not sure how long I did it, but it was for over a year. I know first-hand how much of a huge time investment it is, how much angst it creates, and how it messes with our body signals.

- I've had the experience of finishing my (calorie-budgeted) meal and still being hungry, but feeling like I "couldn't" or wasn't "allowed to" eat more. That feeling is the worst!

- On the flip-side of that, there were times when I'd realize I was done before the meal was over, but I figured I'd just keep eating anyway because I'd already budgeted the calories, and maybe it would prevent me from feeling hungry later.

- The annoyance of measuring out perfectly level tablespoons of peanut butter is something I'm familiar with, unfortunately.

- I know the frustration that is counting all of the calories in every ingredient of a recipe, totaling it all up and dividing by the number of servings to find out how many calories are in each specific serving.

- I'm also familiar with the frustration that then comes when your boyfriend, roommate, husband, or friend takes something bigger or smaller than a perfectly equal serving size. Like, "Nooooo, you just messed up all of my math and now I don't know how much is in my serving!"

- I know how annoying it is to go out to a restaurant and feel intense anxiety because you just have no idea how many calories are in your meal. Either the restaurant doesn't post the calorie info, or you know that the amount of butter your meal is swimming in means that the calorie count they did post was definitely wrong.

- I remember the mental gymnastics that went on when entering my food tallies for the day into my counting software of choice.

  o If my calories were less than the budget, I'd be excited and proud! But then I'd feel like I deserved a cookie for my hard work … and would sometimes eat the cookie even if I wasn't actually hungry, just because the numbers told me I could.

  o If my calories were over budget, my stomach would sink and I'd feel like I messed up or failed.

  o If I found that I'd hit my target allowance for the day, but was still hungry, I had a big decision to make: eat more (and go over my allotted calories and then feel like I failed), or stay hungry so that the numbers end up where they "should" (making me miserable and cranky, and even hungrier when I woke up the next day).

So yeah, I've been there. It's not a fun place to be, and the scenarios above aren't unique to me; they're very common among people who've counted calories (do they resonate with you too?). In these common scenarios, people counting calories are often either suffering through too much hunger because they're "not allowed" to have more food, or they're eating more than they would have if the numbers hadn't told them they had room to eat more.

Counting calories plays mind games with us. It does this on both a meal-to-meal and a day-to-day basis. If we have too many instances of suffering through lots of hunger, we typically end up overeating eventually to finally make that hunger go away (and we subsequently feel bad about it).

If we constantly eat without feeling hungry, even if the numbers say we're allowed to, it's very likely we're taking in more than we actually need, and we won't see the progress that we think we should be making.

For all of these reasons, calorie counting ends up doing more harm than good most times. While it can lead to weight loss when the math really does work out right, it's not the most pleasant way of doing it. And it overshadows our actual relationship with food. We become so focused on the numbers and the data, that we stop enjoying our food.

Is all this effort and hassle worth it? Is the gamble of getting your calorie counts right worth the time it takes to count every calorie? Is it worth the frustration to you and your family as you make decisions based solely on how many calories are in your meals? Is the feeling that you get when the scale disappoints you once again worth the few times that it does line up with what you expect? Is the example you're setting for your kids one that you want to set? When it comes to our overall food relationship, the negatives of counting calories exceed the positives. There is no peace with food here. There is stress, and frustration, and micro-managing, and disappointment.

Getting to a better relationship with our eating takes time, especially when we're coming from a calorie-counting background. It also takes something vitally important that I hope you've started to develop as you've been reading through this book: Trust.

To move away from counting calories, you need to trust yourself. Trust yourself to make decisions that are in your best interest for long-term health and happiness. Trust yourself to be imperfect, because a healthy approach to eating includes being able to eat "imperfectly." Trust yourself to eat like a non-dieter, because you *are* becoming a non-dieter! Trust yourself to be able to find peace with food so that you're not tempted to micro-manage. Finally, trust that you can love yourself as you currently are.

Too Much Hunger

One of the things I mentioned before was the idea of struggling and suffering through lots of hunger. This concept is not unique to calorie counting; it's something many people do in the name of losing weight. I'm willing to bet you've heard some version of the phrase "Hunger is fat cells crying" at some point.

Now, like with many things, there is a nugget of truth in there. If our body needs calories, and we don't give it some, it will burn calories from the stores that we have. This is actually one of the reasons why it's a good idea to avoid snacking between meals. It gives our bodies a chance to practice using those stores, so that our metabolisms are flexible enough to handle situations where food isn't immediately available.

However, more is not always better. It is possible to have too much of a good thing. Just like it is possible to eat too many vegetables and become uncomfortable and bloated, so too is it possible to put yourself through too much hunger so that it backfires.

Enduring hunger for a very long period of time isn't something that tends to be enjoyable for most people. Sure, there are people who practice fasting, and if that's important to you, then I won't tell you to stop. However, if you end the fast by gorging on (and overeating) a ton of food to try to satisfy your pent-up hunger, then I suggest the fast isn't doing you any favors. If any calorie deficit you create by enduring the hunger is obliterated by a massive calorie influx after the fast, you're not accomplishing what you set out to do. And you've only made yourself miserable in the process.

There is a better, easier, less unpleasant way of going about your eating. Paying attention to hunger is important. Eating in response to the bodily cue of hunger is a skill that is very worthy of practice. But there is no need to overdo it. We don't have to manipulate ourselves to work around our hunger. We can listen to it, and honor it. Our bodies will thank us for that.

If we come back to the mindset aspect of all this, it starts to beg the question: Why would you put yourself through too much hunger on purpose? The answer is almost invariably, to lose weight. And we've already discussed how the diet mentality makes us want to lose weight for all the wrong reasons.

If we work on the foundational body image piece of all this, and start to reframe our thinking toward a mentality of "How can I treat myself *better*, and foster *more* health and happiness?", then we realize how making ourselves suffer through endless hunger for no health or happiness benefit doesn't make any sense.

In the next chapter, I'll show you how you can start to make friends with your hunger. It doesn't have to be something you endure for extended periods of time, nor does it have to be something you fear. It is simply a signal, and one which we can start to use as a helpful guide.

The Clean Plate Club

On the flip side of enduring too much hunger is something many of us were taught as children: Clean your plate. This idea is one that has been handed down for generations, and I'm not really sure why. Many of us were told "There are starving kids in Africa," as if that was somehow supposed to make us happily eat more than our bellies actually wanted.

The end result of being taught to clean our plates, or eat everything that is served to us, is that we learn to push past our fullness and satiety signals, and eat more than we actually need.

We start to use the external visual of a clean plate as a cue for knowing when to end a meal, versus the innate ability we were born with to sense our own satiety and stop there.

In a way, it's understandable where this idea may have come from. In times past, when food was scarce, you can bet people finished whatever food they were able to get onto their plates in the first place. We don't live in times of food scarcity anymore, though (at least not most of us). But many people who lived through scarcity carry the remnants of that experience with them. As they grow to raise their own kids in an era of plentiful food, that scarcity is still in the back of their minds, and they encourage cleaning your plate because that's what they had to do when they were young. There is probably also an underlying idea that we should be very grateful for the abundance of food that we now have, since it's not always guaranteed.

But this underlying backstory is lost on children. As kids, all we know is that our belly is full, or we don't like what's on the plate, and we're being forced to eat more when our body is telling us we don't want to.

We started to learn that we shouldn't listen to our bodies, and instead, should be eating to clean the plate, or to make our parents happy, or for some other external reason. This is how we started to move away from our body signals.

If we grew up with a parent who always wanted us to clean our plate, we tend to still carry that habit around with us today. Without thinking too much about it, we plow through the food on our plates, no matter how we feel. For many of us, that habit has led to several instances of feeling very uncomfortable after meals!

And maybe you can't even blame your parents for your Clean Plate Club membership. I was a card-carrying member of the club for years (and it is still something that's challenging for me), but my parents never forced me to clean my plate. I'm not sure if I just followed my dad's example (the man cleans his plate so well my grandfather used to joke that we wouldn't even have to wash it in order to use it again!), or if I just started to do it on my own.

I think that part of it, for me anyway, is that I don't like to waste food. Leaving food on the plate feels wasteful. I know, after working with clients, that I'm not alone in that thinking. Food may be readily accessible to us these days, but many of us are still frugal, or don't want to be wasteful for any number of other reasons. So take heart, my friends. I am right there with you when it comes to not wanting to waste food. But it *is* possible to avoid waste while still honoring our body signals. I'll show you how in the next chapter.

CHAPTER 13: A MORE MINDFUL AND INTUITIVE APPROACH TO EATING

A Preface on Mindfulness

You'll notice that the theme of this chapter, and honestly, an underlying theme of this entire book, is one seemingly simple thing: mindfulness. In order to return to eating in a way that listens to our body signals, we need to pay mindful attention to what those signals are!

Mindfulness gets a bit of a questionable reputation. It conjures images of monks meditating for hours, or yoga retreats full of silence and Zen. While it can certainly be those things (and *is* a big part of them), it doesn't *have* to be.

Mindfulness is something we are all capable of. The most common definition is:

> *"The awareness that emerges through paying attention on purpose, in the present moment, and non-judgmentally to the unfolding of experience moment by moment."*[42]

If I can somehow put it even more simply... it's taking a short time-out from the constant 'go-go-go' of life these days. It's taking a second to breathe, and calm your frazzled mind. Being mindful is incredibly helpful when it comes to this mindset makeover, because so much of the diet mentality has taken hold and become like an autopilot. If we want to change it, we have to start questioning it, and paying attention to the little moments that happen as we go through our day. Now let's dive in and see how this applies to our mindset makeover in terms of tuning in to our body signals.

Learning to Tune In

If you've been ignoring, or even manipulating, your body signals for a while, trying to tune in and be mindful of them may feel uneasy at first, like you don't have a guideline for how to eat. Don't worry, we can still use flexible guidelines to steer our eating to be something that is beneficial to our health and peaceful for our sanity.

While I don't tend to subscribe 100% to any particular way of eating, I do find that many of the things I teach my clients fall closely in line with something called Intuitive Eating. What I outline below is my own take on it.

Step 1: Plan

Planning out your meals does several things:

- It helps that organized side of you feel confident that there is a plan in place so things aren't left 100% to chance.

- It avoids the dreaded "What am I going to make for dinner?" question from being asked every single night.

- It helps you save time and money by only buying what you need at the grocery store, rather than haphazardly taking foods from shelves up and down the aisles, without much planning or thought.

- It allows you to make sure your overall eating for the week contains lots of nutritious foods, and any other less nutritious foods you *want* to include.

If you have a history of calorie counting, that will actually come in handy here at first. Through your counting experience, you've likely become rather familiar with various serving sizes. Start there and use what you know as your guide when planning out your meals. Go back to the Healthy Eating Without Dieting chapter for a refresher on structuring your meals in a sane and healthy way.

Step 2: Tune in *Before* the Meal: Listen for Hunger

Once your meals are planned out, the next step is to wait until you're physically hungry to eat them. Start to tune in and pay mindful attention to that feeling of hunger. What does it feel like? Can you describe it? It may or may not involve the growling stomach noises you think it should!

You don't have to sit with that feeling a long time, but you can start to get reacquainted. Once you've tuned in to that feeling a bit, eat that lovely meal you planned out.

Step 3: Tune in *During* the Meal

As you're eating, take a pause midway through the meal. Tune in. How do you feel? Are you still hungry? Maybe you're not hungry anymore, but you're also not yet satisfied. Whatever you feel, just make a mental note. Don't overthink it, just check to make sure you're not already full!

Step 4: Tune in *After* the Meal

When you finish, tune in again. Was what you served enough? Are you still hungry? Are you too full? Maybe you're just right and totally comfortable? Take stock of how you felt after the meal.

Step 5: Use What You Found to Plan for Future Meals

The info you gather from mindfulness before, during, and after your meal can guide you in your future meal planning and preparation. If it wasn't enough, you know you'll need a little more next time (or if you're able to eat more now so you can get satisfied, go ahead and do that!). If it was too much, you can serve yourself a bit less next time. And if it was just right, give yourself a well-deserved 'high five'!

I find that tuning into hunger (the front-end of the meal) is easier than tuning in and finding the best point at which to stop eating (the back-end of the meal). Don't fret too much about any of it. The biggest take-away here is just to start listening to your body's signals. Once you start listening, you can *then* start to let those signals guide your actions.

Bonus Step 6: Take a Mindfulness Break When Tempted to Eat Emotionally

Taking a quick mindful moment when you're tempted to eat emotionally can help you insert a pause into the autopilot response of dealing with difficult situations with food (which we'll be talking more about in the next section). Taking that moment to get out of autopilot mode means you can *choose* to deal with the situation differently if you'd like to, rather than acting simply on impulse.

We often grab chocolate (or wine) after a stressful day without thinking about it too much. If we insert that short pause, we can make a more conscious choice (and no, that doesn't necessarily mean you have to choose against the chocolate or wine each time!) You just gain back control by giving yourself a moment to think it through.

Calorie Counting Makeover

After reading the previous chapter, I hope you can see the value in moving away from counting calories. Even if you're not counting them to the level of putting them into an app or website tracker, many of us do a bit of mental counting to some extent too. But none of us enjoy it.

If you've been counting calories, macros, or points in some way for a while, I bet it's part of why you're here, doing this work to makeover your diet mentality. Because you know that a desire to count calories is that old diet brain speaking up like the devil on your shoulder.

You want to let your body be your guide, and be able to listen to the hunger and fullness cues your body sends so that you can give your body what it needs without doing so much work! But you're not sure how… So let's discuss how we can start to move in that direction without going completely cold turkey. We're just going to slowly redirect the mindfulness you used to have for calorie counts to your body signals, instead.

Step 1: Start to Listen

You can start to tune in and listen for those body cues while you're still counting, having the counting as a backup plan, instead of the main event. You may still be counting, but when you sit down to eat a meal, insert a bit of mindfulness. Tune in before, during, and after to see if you can hear the cues your body is sending you. Some questions you can ask yourself:

1. Are you actually feeling hunger when the meal starts?
2. Can you notice the hunger lessening as you eat the meal?
3. Are you finding that you feel comfortably satisfied when the meal is over?
4. If not, are you still hungry? Or are you overfull?

Even if you don't change a single thing yet about how you count or how you eat, the simple act of purposely putting your attention onto the body signals is a step in the right direction. This mindfulness in action is a critical first step! Once you're comfortable tuning in and listening (non-judgmentally), you can move on to step 2.

Step 2: Drop *One* Aspect of Counting

This will be the first change made to the actual counting. Pick something to not count or track. Just *one* thing. You can either choose to not count calories for a particular meal (for example: start by not counting calories at lunch anymore, even if you still count at breakfast and dinner), or you can choose to stop tracking one component of your meals (like the veggie portion). The idea is to just start--one small step at a time, and see what it feels like to not count some of your calories. Once you're comfortable here, move on to step 3.

Step 3: Progressively Count Less and Less

Keep making small changes by removing aspects of the counting over time. Perhaps you stop tracking lunches first, then stop tracking breakfasts, then eventually you finally stop tracking dinner too. Maybe you start by not tracking veggies, then move to protein, then to fat, then to carbs.

No matter which way you go about it, keep making small changes that feel doable until you're ready to stop counting all together!

Stop Suffering Through Too Much Hunger

It's absolutely okay to make friends with hunger. If we're going to start working on eating intuitively, part of that is learning to tune in and listen for those hunger signals so we can eat in response to them.

But please remember that more is not always better, and hunger is one area where this is so true. Too much hunger often means that we end up ravenous at our next meal, and have a very difficult time eating mindfully, or stopping before we're overfull.

Make life easier on yourself and learn to be friends with your hunger, rather than enemies. Your hunger is there to guide you. Listen to it, don't purposely ignore it in the name of losing weight.

If you find yourself trying to push off hunger, ask yourself why. Is it logistics or scheduling related, like a meal coming up soon but not immediately? Is it because you're busy and feel like you don't have time to eat now? Is it because you're wanting to lose weight? Your answer to why you're trying to push off your hunger will give you insight into what to do.

Logistics

With logistics, sometimes they just get tricky and we do the best we can to navigate them comfortably. I don't want to say there's any right or wrong way to approach this, but the general premise of honoring your body is what I think should take the lead.

If eating something now (even if you're hungry) means that you won't be hungry for the planned meal that's in an hour, then maybe you'll choose to push it off a bit. Or maybe you'll hold yourself over with something very small, like a few veggies, so you can still feel ready to eat when the meal comes. It's up to you, since you are the one who knows your body best.

Too Busy

If you're feeling like you're too busy to eat, take a moment to get a deep breath and see if it's really 100% true that you can't take a break at all. Sometimes it is true (you're in a meeting you can't get out of, for example), but other times, our perception of our 'busy-ness' is overly inflated. (I'm including myself in this, by the way!)

We are all busy, and I can tell you from experience that there are many things that will take up *all* the time we allow them to. But in the spirit of self-care and our own sanity, we need to put our own needs first sometimes. And I believe that honoring our hunger and giving ourselves the care of a nourishing meal is something we can make time for no matter how busy everything else gets, because when we're happily fed, everything else feels a bit easier.

Weight Loss

Logistics and hectic schedules are things we have to work around sometimes. But please do not push off your hunger in the name of weight loss. If you're tempted to do this, ask yourself if you really want to treat your body this way in order to lose weight. Enduring hunger for a long time is miserable, and it often backfires. Is there a kinder way you can approach it?

Remember that eating before you get overly hungry means you'll have an easier time stopping at a place where you're physically comfortable, versus easily overeating when you're too hungry at mealtime.

This means that when we push hunger off for too long, we actually can end up eating *more* and completely overcompensating for any fat-burning we may have accomplished while we suffered through too much hunger.

If you want to lose weight, find a way to do it that isn't miserable and doesn't backfire on you like fasting or enduring too much hunger does.

Leaving the Clean Plate Club Behind

As someone who has always cleaned the plate even though no one actually taught me to, I know how hard it is to try to change this habit. Many of our clients have trouble with this idea at first.

There are two ways I typically approach this with clients:

- Serve less food to begin with
- Practice leaving a bite or two behind

Option 1: Serve Less Food

The first method tends to be easier for many people (me included). If you don't like to waste food, then it makes sense to serve yourself a portion that is closer to the amount you'll actually eat. Yes, the amount your body needs is likely slightly different on a day-to-day basis, which is why tuning in is still a necessary skill to work on. But I find it's always best to make things as easy for yourself as possible. Why serve yourself a pound of spaghetti on a huge plate and then try to figure out when to stop? It's much easier to serve a smaller amount, eat that, then decide how you feel and if you need or want more.

Option 2: Practice Leaving 1-2 Bites

The second option, practicing leaving bites behind, is tougher but also extremely valuable. Again, I'm not a fan of wasting food if I can help it. However, leaving one bite of food on the plate feels pretty doable. Rationally, we know in our minds that the calories in that one tiny bite aren't likely to make a huge difference in how we feel or how long that meal keeps us satisfied. And throwing one bite of food in the trash isn't very wasteful either. So this exercise is a really great way to practice chipping away at the visual cue of a clean plate to end the meal with. One bite, that's it.

And a helpful tidbit: it doesn't have to be the best bite. What I mean by that is, if you're having a meal that you love, but there is one piece of potato that got a bit too crispy, or a veggie that got a bit soggy, or a too-chewy piece of chicken. Leave that bite. You won't miss it, I promise. You don't have to leave the most tender bite of filet mignon on your plate, you can leave the soggy zucchini slice, instead. Leaving one bite is, of course, only the first step. It's not really the end goal. What is the goal?

The Ultimate Goal: Use How You *Feel* as the Cue to Stop Eating

The idea is to work your way up to becoming comfortable leaving more than one bite. Ideally, we want to start to become comfortable ending the meal based only on how we feel, not based on what's left on the plate. This can mean no bites left, or half a meal left, depending on what was on the plate to begin with.

At home, it's pretty easy to leave one bite, or a couple bites. When we go out to dinner at a restaurant, though, portions tend to be rather huge. In this situation, leaving only one bite may still leave you feeling stuffed, so you'll want some other ideas to help you manage those epic portions and stop eating before you feel stuffed.

Restaurant Strategies That Can Help

- Order small plates, like appetizers. Often, the appetizers are large enough to be a full meal. Pairing an appetizer with a side of veggies is often a great size for a meal that is likely to get you satisfied without feeling stuffed.

- Swap veggies for a heavier side. Many menu items come with potatoes or french fries as a side. See if you can swap it with something lighter, more nutritious, and less likely to leave you stuffed.

- Ask for a take-out container at the start of the meal. This is one of the oldest tricks in the book, but it does help tremendously to put some of the meal out of sight and out of mind. This is a way of essentially helping the restaurant serve you less (and as a bonus, you get a meal for tomorrow too!).

- Check in with your stomach periodically. Put the fork down, take a sip of water, or chat with your companions for a moment. Insert a mindful pause during your meal so that you can take a moment to tune in and see how you feel. If you're still hungry, keep eating. If you're comfortably satisfied, stop and ask for a take-out container. If you're already overfull, don't keep eating even more.

These are just a few ways you can start to step away from the Clean Plate Club. As always, this skill takes practice. You don't do it a new way once and never have a hard time with overeating again. Many clients work on this skill for a very long time, and honestly, I think most of us are constantly working on practicing this, because it's hard! But put in the practice to start chipping away at that Clean Plate Club mentality, because it will serve you well in the long run and go a long way in helping you to ditch the diet mindset. (Because when we overeat, we tend to start thinking about how we'll restrict or diet tomorrow, don't we?)

CHAPTER 14: ENCOURAGING MINDFUL AND INTUITIVE EATING IN KIDS

Now that we've discussed a makeover to our own approach to eating – using body signals instead of calorie counts, plate visuals, or suffering through too much hunger – it's time to chat about how we can set our kids up for success in this area as well. First, I'll tell you about some of the very common things most of us say and do when eating with our kids that have the unintended effect of steering them away from their body signals. Then we'll get into how to revise our approach to encourage mindfulness and honoring those body signals!

How We Inadvertently Guide Our Kids Away from Their Body Signals

Every time we talk to our kids about food, we are helping to shape how they approach it. There are phrases and ideas that we communicate to them that may not have the intended message we mean to give them. For example, when we tell them to eat two more bites of something after they've declared that they're done, we are guiding them away from their satiety signals. Bribing them to finish their broccoli by promising dessert does the same thing, and it *also* suggests that the dessert is a reward for getting through the punishment of eating the broccoli (not really the message most of us are trying to send).

Believe me, I know we're all just trying to get our kids to eat well. We watch them eat only the bread and try to find creative ways to get them to at least try the other stuff on their plate too. It's incredibly tempting, and I know I've done it myself. But we do them a disservice if we steer them away from their hunger and fullness in the process, using phrases like the ones below:

- "Two more bites, then you can be excused."
- "You didn't eat much, have more of your chicken."
- "You can't be hungry, you just ate!"
- "If you eat more broccoli, we can have a cookie after dinner."
- "That's enough, you've eaten a lot already."

These statements can lead to overriding kids' inner body signals and suggest that they need to listen to us (or some other external stimulus) to know how much to eat.

Encouraging a More Intuitive and Mindful Approach

How can we approach things a bit differently in order to keep the focus on helping our kiddos tune into, and honor, their body signals? The general idea is to phrase our comments and questions to them in ways that bring the focus back onto those signals.

Keep in mind, there is an age appropriateness to this idea. When kids are little, it's difficult to know when they are able to accurately assess their body signals.

Babies do it pretty instinctively, plus they're only eating (drinking) one food source for the first few months, so taste preferences don't really play much of a role. But as kids get older, and they start to eat actual foods, and they develop likes and dislikes, and we start to use phrases like the ones in the above section, things start to get a bit confusing.

We need to remember that we are the sidekick to their body signal guides. We help by providing structure, variety, and opportunity to their eating, while encouraging them to eat how their bodies guide them.

Structure

Having a flexible structure to meals and snacks is immensely helpful in developing a routine to your day. After a while, it also helps kids' appetites to regulate a bit so they're hungry around the times that food is served.

One of the keys to ensuring that kids are actually hungry at meals and snacks is to avoid grazing and nibbling (and drinking things other than water) between these times. If we allow them to constantly graze and nibble, it makes the lines between hungry and full harder to differentiate. Allowing them to develop actual hunger before eating times means they're better able to understand what the feeling is and what it means.

While structure is good, we still like to approach it as guidelines. Sometimes the meal times are flexible, like at home on the weekends, and we can shift things back or forward depending on hunger. Other times, meals need to be at certain times (think of daycare and school schedules where meals and snacks are fixed).

So, like with so many things in life, we find a balance. We don't want to leave all meals and snacks up to our kids' hunger, which can be unpredictable. But we also don't want to force them to eat when "it's time for lunch." So we encourage listening in for those signals and eating in accordance with them. But we also have to set limits somewhere so that they don't refuse lunch only to demand a snack 10 minutes later.

That sounds complicated when it's written out like that, but if you think about it, we do this with ourselves all the time. When we're at work, we typically have a set lunch time. We also usually need to eat breakfast at a certain time before leaving for work, and then dinner tends to have to be a certain time so the kids can get to bed on time too.

We have a routine, and if we want to let our signals be our guides, we try to reverse engineer our hunger so we get hungry at the times we need to be eating. On weekends, when the routine is less structured, we can be a bit more flexible and follow our signals more directly. However, if we're pretty accustomed to a routine, it'll usually end up still fitting pretty close to that general timeframe. It's the same for kids. So determine a routine and flexible structure to meal/snack times that work for your family, and then go from there!

Phrases That Help

Once you have a general routine in mind, the idea is to guide things so that hunger is present for those meal and snack times. Sometimes you'll nail it, and you and the kids will be hungry for the meal and eat enough to stay comfortable until the next meal.

But appetites, especially in kids, can be wonky. They're not always consistent, and sometimes they won't be hungry for a meal, or they'll be super hungry way too early. This is why flexibility is a good thing. But we also need to still have a boundary somewhere so they're not grazing between meals and hampering their hunger for the next meal.

There's no magic formula to making this work perfectly (because really, life never works out "perfectly," does it?). But here are some phrases you can use to encourage a focus on body signals while keeping with a flexible structure:

- You seem like you're all done eating/you're not hungry anymore. Should I put the rest of your food away for later? (For when they're done at a meal even if they barely ate... a replacement for the "two more bites, please" we usually say!)

- It's just about snack time. Are you hungry now, or do you want to wait a couple of minutes? (For those times when things are more flexible.)

- If you're not hungry, you don't need to eat now. Just remember we won't have snack for another two hours. (For times when things aren't as flexible.)

- Is your belly hungry, or are you looking for something fun to do? (For when you think they might be confusing hunger with boredom.)

Balancing Real Hunger and Taste Hunger

There is a potential trap that we can fall into when we start putting emphasis on hunger, which I think is important to watch out for. Dr. Dina Rose says that when we focus *too* much on asking kids to only eat when they're hungry, they actually learn to… Wait for it… Lie.[43]

They'll say "I'm hungry" when really they just saw a yummy cookie that they want. They'll say "I'm not hungry" if they don't like what is served for a meal, or if they'd rather keep playing with whatever they're currently doing.

Man, we parents can't catch a break, can we?! As Dina points out, there are a couple different types of hunger outside of true physical hunger: Taste Hunger and Emotional Hunger.[43] We'll address the emotional hunger piece in the Emotional Eating section, but I think it's super noteworthy to discuss taste hunger here.

Kids aren't the only ones who experience this. We do it too. Have you ever eaten a nice dinner, stopping when you were comfortably satisfied… and then someone brought out dessert? "Hmm, that dessert looks pretty yummy, I want some!" you think to yourself.

If we want to eat purely for physical hunger alone, we are left with a conundrum… we "can't" eat it because we're not physically hungry anymore! But here again is why this isn't about rules, or doing something "perfectly" 100% of the time. While we don't want to give in to taste hunger every time, I think it's reasonable to *mindfully* indulge in it occasionally. This is true for both us and our kids.

We want to encourage listening to and honoring actual hunger and fullness signals the majority of the time. But we don't want to force our kids to tell us they're hungry in order to be allowed to eat a cupcake!

I find that taste hunger seems to happen most often in relation to less-nutritious foods like desserts. Those foods are ones that we tend to eat primarily because they taste good, not for their nutritional value. And here is where the boundaries you decided on in the good/bad foods section come into play. You (or your kids) may not be physically hungry anymore when the dessert comes out, but you can tune in to how you feel (are you already overfull?), keep your less-nutritious food boundaries in mind, and make a choice to either have some dessert or not.

With kids, we can help them keep to a reasonable portion, as opposed to an all-out sweetsfest, and encourage them to stop eating if their belly starts to feel uncomfortable. It's not about the sweets. It's about avoiding physical discomfort from overeating, regardless of whatever they're overeating.

SECTION 5: EMOTIONAL EATING

CHAPTER 15: EATING IS NOT THE ONLY WAY TO MANAGE EMOTIONS

Eating to manage emotions is something that is so incredibly common, and so seemingly universal, that we even joke about it. We talk about diving into a gallon of ice cream when going through a bad break up, or de-stressing from a busy day with a few glasses of wine. There are even shirts, mugs, and socks out there that poke fun at how often we use chocolate or wine to get through life. This concept of using food to deal with emotions is so prevalent that it's considered the norm. It's not just the negative emotions that are met with food, either. We also use food to celebrate, and to reward ourselves.

All of these things are fine to do periodically, when we actively choose to do them because we truly want to, and we're okay with doing so. As the saying goes: "If it ain't broke, don't fix it." Food is joyful, and can have its place when it comes to helping us feel good.

However, if food is the only tool at your disposal when emotions get tricky, then eating for emotions can often become something that is only enjoyable in the short term. It is very commonly met with regret later on, either because it makes a person feel physically unwell, or because they feel guilty.

Eating for Negative Emotions

While there are a myriad of negative emotions that fall under this heading (stress, sadness, boredom, anger, frustration, disappointment, etc.), at the very core, people seem to be looking for an escape. We just want to not feel bad anymore.

That makes total sense, doesn't it? Who wants to feel bad? No one I know! When we are feeling a way we don't want to feel, we look for a way out, a way to feel better right this very moment. And most of us turn to food.

Why do we use food to feel better? We do that because it does feel like it works in the short term. It provides a couple of minutes of enjoyment so that we can mentally check out of the negative space we were just in. We get to enjoy a little oasis in the middle of a vast desert of difficulty, and it feels nice in that moment.

Researchers have a few ideas as to why we turn to eating, or overeating/bingeing, when we're facing negative emotions:

- We do it to escape uncomfortable self-awareness by shifting our attention onto something else.[44] It distracts us, and allows us to "avoid dealing with ego-threatening information."[45]

- We like the pleasurable experience of eating, or we like eating "bad" foods that we're usually not allowing ourselves to eat.[45]

- We do it in an attempt to shift the blame for the negativity away from the true cause and onto the eating itself.[2] It's easier to blame our bad feelings on our overeating or our food choices than on what's really going on.

So we do it to escape, and to feel better in the short-term. But when we stop eating, do we still feel better? Usually, the answer is no. And sometimes, we feel even worse because we realize we just ate more than we needed and we don't feel good about that, either physically or mentally. Feeling worse certainly isn't what we were going for! So we start to find ourselves in another cycle:

Emotional Eating Cycle

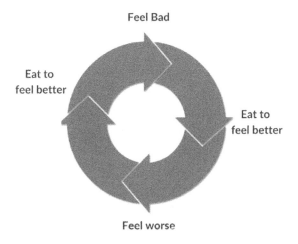

Feel Bad

Eat to feel better

Eat to feel better

Feel worse

The moral of the story here is that emotional eating doesn't actually help us feel better. It is a sign that we are having difficulty managing our emotions. Essentially, using food is a crutch when we feel unable to deal with emotions directly.

Eating for Emotion Management Doesn't Do Us Any Favors

Eating emotionally doesn't promote our overall health. "In adults and adolescents, emotional eating has been linked to heavier weight, obesity, and greater consumption of energy-dense sweet and salty foods."[46]

Both chronic dieters and people with obesity have a greater tendency to use food in reaction to negative emotions. But it is certainly not limited to those populations, as it's been seen in healthy, non-dieting people as well.[45]

It's not the negative emotions themselves that lead to emotional eating; it's the inability to regulate and deal with those emotions that leads us to eat or overeat in reaction.[45] And this tendency to eat for emotions is then correlated to a higher incidence of overweight and obesity.

To sum it up, emotional eating is a short-term distraction from negative feelings that can impact our long-term health, especially if we do it often. And in this way, it comes back to an idea we mentioned in the self-kindness and self-compassion chapter: that there is a difference between short-term indulgence and long-term kindness.

Eating to squash an emotion feels nice in the moment, and we can almost convince ourselves that it's the kind thing to do, or a way of treating ourselves well. But if doing so can be associated with long-term consequences to our health, is it really the best way to keep both our health *and* happiness in mind?

Can We Stop Eating for Emotions?

If we want to stop the cycle of feel bad → eat → feel worse → eat, we have to start doing something differently. And the very first step in this process is simply this: We have to be open to the idea that something other than food can help.

That sounds like super "Captain Obvious" stuff, but it's surprising how often we don't consider that there are viable alternatives out there. Food has worked, temporarily, in the past, so we continue to do it. And we tend to also continue not really liking that decision after the fact. So the first step in stopping this emotional eating cycle is to be open to the possibility of an alternative. Not just an alternative either... but a *better* alternative. One that works in both the short term and the long term.

Ultimately, if the core of emotional eating is not being able to regulate our emotions very well, we can learn to respond to those more effectively. "Although it may sometimes be impossible to avoid experiencing negative emotions, it may be possible (though perhaps complicated) to change the way we regulate these emotions and thereby remove an important instigator of emotional eating."[45]

Eating for Reward or Celebration

"I deserve a cookie after that long run."

"Let's go out for ice cream to celebrate!"

"I ate clean all week, so today is my cheat day."

Do these things sound familiar? If so, then you're probably familiar with the idea of eating, or eating certain things, for the sake of celebration or reward. We all do it. It's customary to celebrate birthdays with cake, after all! But doing this too often, or celebrating every little accomplishment with a food reward, starts to lead down a tricky path. We start to give food powers it doesn't have, and we start to see it as a catch-all reward or celebration solution.

Celebration Eating

If you think about it, we seem to be able to find "special occasions" in just about anything nowadays. Going to the movies, catching a baseball game, date night with our loved one, and pretty much every weekend are causes to celebrate.

I think it's important to point out that eating *is* an enjoyable thing to do. It's pleasurable. And we can certainly celebrate and eat without it being a problem at all. Hey, when food is delicious, every meal is its own celebration!

However, when most of us celebration-eat, it typically means overeating and/or eating more less-nutritious foods than usual. We start to use celebrations as an excuse to eat in a way that doesn't really line up with our values of eating to promote our long-term health and happiness.

Think of things like Thanksgiving, where it's considered the norm to overeat to the point of discomfort. (We joke about needing elastic waistbands for this epic meal, right?)

Think of the sweets that have become associated with the various holidays or times of year (pumpkin spice everything, peppermint mochas, candies at Easter, Halloween, and Valentine's Day, etc.).

Think of how various foods, particularly the less-nutritious ones, get associated with simple activities like going to the movies (popcorn drowned in butter), watching our kids' sports games (ice cream, hot dogs, and candy), or fundraising (bake sales galore).

There is absolutely nothing wrong with celebrating things in life. In fact, I think celebrating the little things is something we could all do *more* of! But celebrating doesn't have to mean overeating or eating lots of less-nutritious foods. We can celebrate and enjoy life without always attaching it to eating that way. If we want to build and maintain a positive and healthy relationship with food, part of that means lessening our dependence on foods for enjoyment.

The moral of the story here is that foods, and more specifically the less-nutritious foods, don't have to be the primary way in which we celebrate things.

They can certainly be part of the overall picture (because again, we're not making rules here to say that we can never celebrate with food). But finding other ways to celebrate means we keep a positive food relationship intact, and we also open our horizons to other enjoyable celebration possibilities!

Food as Reward

There will always be things in life that we don't really want to do. It might be picking up an extra shift at work when someone is out, or doing a workout when you'd rather stay in bed at 5am, or driving your mom to the airport. There are a bazillion things in life that we don't necessarily *want* to do, especially at the time. But we do them. And sometimes, we feel like we deserve something in return for doing something we weren't really all too keen on doing.

Enter the food reward. I see this idea tied to workouts a lot, since many of my clients are interested in fitness. There is something in many peoples' minds that says a hard workout gets rewarded with food. I'm not sure where this came from. Yes, working out hard means you burned more calories than if you sat around doing nothing. Food is inevitably tied to working out because hard work *does* require more fuel. That's just a physical reality.

But your body will increase its hunger accordingly, and we can simply listen to it in order to adjust our intake in the way our body needs.

Going for a long run or hitting the weights for an hour doesn't mean you "earned" food or sweets, though. Nor do we earn it for getting through anything else that was tough, difficult, or just not fun. Food isn't a reward. It's just food. As my good friend and mentor Georgie Fear says: "You wouldn't think you deserve to wear yellow today, would you? So why would you deserve less healthy food after a particularly hard day at the office?"

What Are We Really Looking For?

When we are looking for a reward, it usually means we have something to do that's not very pleasurable, and we want to balance that out with something that *is* pleasurable. That makes total sense, because we all want to enjoy life and not have our days disproportionately filled with things we don't like.

But just like food doesn't have to be tied to every celebration, it also doesn't need to be the only way in which we balance the scales of fun/not-fun.

Food is enjoyable, absolutely. And there is nothing wrong with this. I don't want this section to come across as a suggestion that we should never eat for pleasure or enjoyment, and should only view food as a fuel. It is both! We can't ignore the aspects of eating that are outside of pure fuel, because that's not reality!

The key, though, is to be mindful of the reasons we eat, and to balance them so that we're not overly turning to food for pleasure-seeking. As psychotherapist Tabitha Limotte says:

> *"Food is emotional and pleasurable. It evokes memories, connects us to each other, and it soothes. It is also the fuel that operates our bodies and minds. A mindful approach toward eating has to operate within this tension.*
>
> *"The danger comes when we take extreme views toward food. For example, saying to yourself that you have to 'earn' the right to eat by finishing tasks, exercising, dieting heavily, or by relying on food as the only source of relief from emotions."*[47]

In the next chapter, I'll give you what I call my "Emotional Eating Toolkit." It is a series of non-food tools that you can add to your emotions management toolbox, so that food no longer has to be the default setting in responding to emotions.

CHAPTER 16: NON-FOOD STRATEGIES FOR MANAGING EMOTIONS

Before we get into the meat of this chapter, please remember that we're not replacing old rules with new rules. This is not a "do not ever use food for emotions" kind of thing. This is simply an avenue through which we give ourselves other options, so that we have a whole toolbox of things to choose from when facing various emotions.

If we want to start rewiring our brains to avoid automatically turning to food when life gets tough, the first order of business, before we even get to the new tools, is a simple three-step process: Pause, Identify, Accept.

Pause → Identify → Accept

1. The PAUSE is necessary to interrupt the automatic response of 'feel bad = eat something.' Since this is a habit that we've probably had for a very long time, we need to disrupt the autopilot response if we want to attempt something different.

2. Once we've paused, what do we do next? We IDENTIFY the emotion by asking ourselves: What am I actually feeling right now? Many times, I think we start to lump all the negative stuff under the umbrella of feeling "bad." But emotions are more nuanced than that, and different emotions may require different solutions. So take that pause to figure out specifically what it is you're struggling with.

3. The next step is to ACCEPT that feeling. Succinctly put: It's okay to feel bad sometimes. Humans experience a huge range of emotions, and not all of them are positive ones. That is okay, and it's absolutely normal. We can't feel happy and excited 24/7. That's not real life! So one of the biggest ways we can help ourselves cope with the negative emotions is to accept that they are part of normal, chaotic, everyday life.

Once you start to accept that it's okay to feel bad sometimes, then you have four options to choose from to deal with situations compassionately:

1. Find a way to address it or fix it
2. Let it pass on its own
3. Choose to let it go
4. Cope with it to feel better

I find that there are usually two main pathways for negative or difficult emotions. As you can see in the graphic that follows, they diverge with a simple question: Is the cause of this feeling something I can directly act on to either fix the problem or address the underlying need?

Response Options to Negative Emotions

```
┌──────────────────────────┐
│  Feel something negative │
└──────────────────────────┘
             │
             ▼
┌──────────────────────────┐
│ Accept that you feel that way │
└──────────────────────────┘
             │
             ▼
┌──────────────────────────┐
│   Can I fix this directly? │
└──────────────────────────┘
      (Yes)        (No)
      ↙               ↘
┌────────────────┐  ┌──────────────────────────┐
│ 1) Fix/address it │  │ 2) Let it pass on its own │
└────────────────┘  │ 3) Choose to let it go    │
                    │ 4) Cope to feel better    │
                    └──────────────────────────┘
```

Toolkit Option 1 – Address or Fix It

If the answer to whether or not the cause of our negative feelings can be addressed directly is yes, we know there is a specific thing that can help to actually get rid of the cause of our negative emotion.

- If we're angry at someone, we can talk with them and resolve the issue.

- If we're lonely, we can call a friend to talk.

- If we're bored, we can find something to do that we enjoy.

- If we're tired and cranky, we can rest, nap, or go to bed earlier.

- If we're overwhelmed by too many plans, we can say no to some to gain back some free time.

These things all have something that directly addresses the underlying emotion. Once the cause is taken care of, we tend to feel better!

For many of us, our default action for all of the things above is food (or wine). But taking a moment to mindfully assess the feeling and determine if it has a "fix" means we're able to feel better faster, and the underlying issue doesn't remain unresolved like it would if we distracted ourselves temporarily with food. It's a win-win!

If the feeling doesn't have an underlying cause that can be directly addressed, then we move on to the other three options…

Toolkit Option 2 – Let It Pass On Its Own

Have you ever considered the possibility that you don't actually have to *do* anything to make a bad feeling go away? Believe me, as silly as that question sounds, it kind of floored me the first time I heard it. You mean I don't have to escape it, hide from it, or try to fix it? Wow, I'd never thought of that! And once someone draws back the curtain on that possibility, suddenly it's like we have permission to let ourselves feel that way because we know it isn't forever. And that is very freeing.

In a way, this comes back to mindfulness. We allow ourselves to be present with this emotion, even if it's not a positive one, because we know it's a normal human feeling and it will pass in time. Just because we feel sad, lonely, or angry right now, doesn't mean we will still feel that way in an hour, or in a day. It's that age-old cliché: **"This too shall pass."**

I use that as a little mantra sometimes when I'm caught up in an emotion and find myself wanting to eat or otherwise escape it. "This too shall pass" seems to help take some of the urgency out of the feeling.

Dismiss the urge to do something. I know that when we feel bad, we get urges to do something about it. But we don't always have to act on those urges, especially if that urge is for something unhelpful (like eating).

When we get an urge to do something that another part of us doesn't want to do, it can be helpful to dismiss that urge. We do this all the time with non-food urges like:

- Punching your boss when he demands mandatory overtime
- Calling in sick every day that you don't want to go to work
- Telling off your in-laws for making a stupid comment
- Purposely rear-ending the rude driver who cut you off

In each of these, we get an urge to do something based on some type of negative stimulus. We can't really control the urge from happening--it just happens automatically. But we *can* control how we respond to it.

- We don't punch our boss because we'd get fired, or even arrested.
- We don't call in sick every day because we'd be out of a job and we need to make money to support our family.

- We don't tell off our in-laws because it's important to keep the peace, for everyone's sake.
- We don't hit the car who cut us off because we don't want to pay for repair bills or medical treatment if anyone got hurt.

These urges that happen betray one of our other values, and we realize that acting on the urge won't help us in the long run. In these situations, we're able to keep the long-term values in perspective enough to prevent ourselves from acting on the short-term impulse that would feel good for a minute, but would lead to regret later on.

Eating to manage emotions is the same thing. It's an urge that happens, partially due to previous habit in this case. It's fine for the urge to come up. But we are not a slave to it, and we do not have to listen to it. We can find another outlet for our feelings, either by letting it pass, or by finding a more productive way to cope.

Toolkit Option 3 – Choose to Let It Go

If we can't find a direct fix for our problem, and we don't want to wait for it to pass on its own, we have two more options left, both of which can help us to feel better.

Option 3 is to take a cue from Elsa and *Let It Go*. Letting it go seems to always be easier said than done. The first time it was suggested to me I totally scoffed at the idea. How was I supposed to just stop being angry?

It comes back to mindfulness and choice. If there is nothing we can do to fix the thing that upset us, we can choose to let it go. It may be simple, but that doesn't mean it's easy. It takes practice, like anything else.

Sometimes I like to use a little visual imagery to help me let go of something that I can't fix. If you'll indulge a Harry Potter reference for a minute, I like to think of the negative feeling or emotion like one of the memories in Dumbledor's Pensieve. If you have no idea what I'm talking about, let me explain...

He points his wand to his temple, and draws out a memory from his mind. In the movie, it looks like a little wisp of white, glowing smoke. He then empties this memory into a Pensieve to save it and protect it. The thought no longer takes up space in his mind.

My version is slightly different, but the imagery works. Imagine drawing the negative emotion out of you like the little wisp of smoke. Once it's out of your mind, you can acknowledge it, and then rather than save it, let that little puff of smoke dissipate into the air... effectively letting it go. By letting it go, it no longer takes up your prime mental real estate, and you can move on.

Perhaps you're starting to think I'm a bit nutty to suggest this, or to use so many movie references in one chapter, but I think you'll find this is applicable to many of life's little frustrations (and can certainly be used on bigger frustrations too).

Here are some examples of things that bother us, but that we can't change:

- Anger at the very rude driver who cut us off
- Disappointment when the restaurant was out of our favorite menu item
- Frustration after a stressful day at work (like when the boss demanded mandatory overtime!)

These things are ones that we can't change, and holding onto our anger, disappointment, or frustration only causes us to wallow in a negative state. Instead, we can choose to accept our feeling, and then release it, and let it go. The mental exercise of removing the negativity from our minds is powerful enough to help us feel better without doing anything else.

Try this… close your eyes and ask yourself "Since I can't change this, can I at least try to allow myself to let this anger/frustration/stress go?"

If you can answer "yes" to that, then imagine pulling the feeling out of your mind to release it. Or maybe imagine rolling it up into a ball and throwing it away. Find the imagery that works for you. (And don't forget to take a deep breath –it helps!) If we can't just let it go, then we move on to the last option: Finding a way to cope.

Toolkit Option 4 – Find a Non-Food Way to Feel Better

Here, we finally get to the option of doing something to help ourselves feel better. Food is the default most of us are used to, but as I mentioned earlier, we can be open to the possibility that other things can work just as well, if not better.

Ideally, we choose something that not only works in the short term, but also keeps our long-term health and happiness in mind. Think of things that make you happy. When we're feeling low, these things can help us feel better and get us out of our bad mood. Not only do they help when we're in the middle of a tough emotion, but they can also work as a preventative measure. Doing things that add joy to our lives makes us more resilient to the inevitable bad things that happen. When our happiness cup is full, it makes the difficult experiences in life easier to weather.

Below is a list of some generally enjoyable things that serve both of these purposes – filling your happiness cup in general, and ways to cheer yourself up when you're feeling low. A list of enjoyable things to do will be different for each person, of course. I personally wouldn't choose to knit or garden if I wanted to feel better, since those aren't enjoyable for me. However, they might work wonders for someone else.

- Reading for fun
- Taking a bubble bath
- Going for a walk outside
- Dancing (Random dance parties in the kitchen are a mainstay at my house!)
- Taking a hike
- Getting cozy on the couch with a blanket and a cup of tea (bonus if there's a fireplace involved!)
- Petting your dog/cat
- Coloring or drawing

- Listening to music
- Playing an instrument
- Playing a game (board game, video game, whatever)
- Watching a movie
- Watching TV
- Swimming
- Shopping
- Gardening
- Sewing/knitting
- Meditating/Praying
- Journaling
- Singing
- Puzzles (jigsaw, Sudoku, crosswords, etc.)
- Playing with your kids
- Going to a park
- Exercise/yoga/stretching
- Lighting a scented candle
- Calling a friend
- Getting engaged in a project
- Scrapbooking
- Watching the sunset
- Lying down to just breathe
- Looking through pictures (on your phone, in albums, of past vacations, etc.)

I encourage you to create your own list. Pull the ones from this list that interest you, and then think of other things that make *you* happy. Creating a list of only things you personally enjoy means that you'll have a bunch of options available to refer back to the next time you're tempted to eat for emotions.

The idea is two-fold: First, use these things to elevate your background level of happiness before tough emotions come up. Second, start to take a pause when that temptation to eat emotionally starts to happen. In that pause, refer to your list and pick something to try before going for the food.

Even if you still choose the food for a while, you'll be starting to break the automatic response and allow yourself to realize that other options are available. Eventually, you may find that you prefer trying some of these options instead, because they work both in the short term and in the long term.

Celebration and Reward – Adding Non-Food Joy

Food tastes good. Newsflash, right? And food that is hyper-palatable (high in sugar and/or fat and usually also less nutritious) tends to taste really good. In today's world food is everywhere, and we find ourselves rewarding ourselves (and our kids) with food or drinks more often than we probably realize.

Got a promotion at work? Break out the bubbly! Survived a tough day? Get out some wine, and maybe some chocolate. Made it through a tough workout? Have some pizza, you earned it! Kids finally in bed, and the house is tidy for once? Celebrate with a chocolate mug cake!

We all do it to some extent. And as was mentioned before, to a point it's normal! Birthday cake at a birthday party isn't something anyone would find out of place. It's the idea that we "earn" food, or can "reward" ourselves with certain foods that can be problematic, especially if we do it often.

So what can we do instead? Again, the recurring theme comes into play: mindfulness. Being aware of these reward and celebration thought patterns is the first step in being able to makeover that mindset. Then we can start to reframe those thoughts into more constructive ones. Instead of "I deserve to eat _____," what do you really deserve and want?

We deserve to relax.

We deserve to feel happy.

We deserve to treat ourselves well.

We deserve to be cared for.

We deserve some fun.

Once we see what it is we actually want and deserve, we can see how food doesn't always fit the bill, nor is it usually the best or most effective option. Focusing on this means we get to let some other ideas come to the forefront, so we can truly enjoy the things we really want!

In the spirit of treating our bodies well for both health and happiness, especially in the long term, it's a great idea to find some non-food ways of rewarding ourselves and celebrating too, so we can take the focus off the food, and onto the enjoyment! So the next time you're tempted to automatically celebrate something or reward yourself with food, think about what you actually want and deserve.

Here are some examples: If you had to wake up before dawn to drive your mom to the airport, you probably want (and deserve) a nap! If you had a rough and hectic week, you probably want and deserve some time to yourself to relax! Think of some of the things you've been turning to food to reward yourself with, and see if you can find the underlying thing you're really wanting.

Toolkit Option 5: Non-Food Rewards and Ways to Add Joy

When it comes to finding non-food ways to add joy, they can often be similar to the list I included in the last toolkit option (non-food ways to feel better). If you look closely, though, you'll notice that some of these are a little different. Some of the enjoyable things on the previous list may not feel very celebratory, whereas more of the options on this list might seem better aligned with celebrations.

Similarly to the previous list, this is all about finding things that will work well in your own personal toolkit. Use this list as a starting point to get some ideas, then add ones you like that aren't listed to create your own! Here are some non-food ways to reward yourself, celebrate, and also just generally add more joy to your life:

- Date night with your partner (doesn't have to include food)
- Massage
- Manicure/Pedicure/Facial
- Fun new experience, like an Escape Room
- Let grandma take the kids overnight so you can sleep in! (And enjoy coffee in peace for once!)

- Take a nap
- Do a movie night at home
- Plan a vacation
- Go on vacation, even if just for a weekend somewhere close by
- Buy something special
- Do something nostalgic, like bowling or roller skating
- At-home spa day/evening
- Bubble bath with candles
- Read an awesome new book
- Get out in nature
- Go to a zoo or aquarium
- Have a board game night with friends
- Do a puzzle
- Cuddle in front of a fireplace (by yourself, with a loved one, or with a pet, they're all fun!)
- See a play
- Go to a concert
- Find a free event nearby
- Go to a local festival

I hope this chapter has given you some new tools for your emotional management toolbox. Eating to manage emotions is a very difficult thing to stop, and it takes time and practice to start incorporating other things. But it is a very valuable thing to do!

CHAPTER 17: AVOIDING FOOD REWARDS/ EMOTIONAL EATING IN KIDS

Have you ever tried to bribe your kid to eat their veggies by promising dessert after dinner? Have you ever used food as a reward for learning a behavior, like potty training or doing chores? Or maybe the opposite happens and kids aren't allowed to have their favorite treat if they misbehave?

If so, don't worry, you are definitely not alone! This is an amazingly common way we stressed-out parents try to help our kids grow into healthy and responsible humans. It's very likely our parents did this with us, and it seems to work for lots of people, so why not give it a go, right?

This approach seems to work great on the surface. The parents use a reward (something yummy) to get the child to do something (read, do chores, go to the potty, eat more vegetables, etc.). The child does it, which makes the parent happy, and the kid gets something yummy, which makes the kid happy. So it's just one big win-win, right? Not really.

Using Food as a Reward Can Have Unintended Consequences

If we take a moment to step back from the short-term view and see the bigger picture, we realize that this approach is starting to teach some things we aren't really meaning to teach[46,48–50]:

- It can suggest that sweets or other less-nutritious foods are akin to prizes or privileges that can be either earned or taken away.

- It means less-nutritious foods are offered more often, and make up a higher proportion of kids' overall eating pattern.

- It can hint to them that vegetables are just foods to suffer through in order to "earn" sweet foods.

- It can link unpleasant experiences to coping or rewarding with food, especially less-nutritious food.

- It actually *increases* their preference for high-fat and high-sugar foods.[51]

- It can encourage kids to eat when they're not hungry, just to reward themselves.

- It encourages overeating by having them eat more vegetables to earn (and then also eat) dessert.

"When young children are given a treat for a certain behavior, a task, or their eating performance, they learn that the reward of food (often a dessert) is more important than the behavior, task, or food eaten in the first place. Food rewards have the power to shift a child's food value system to favoring sweets or other treats over healthy food. Often, this is opposite of what parents are trying to achieve."[50]

Using food as a reward with kids is a short-term focus that doesn't keep the end game of raising a healthy human with a healthy food relationship in mind.

Moving Away from Food Rewards with Kids

This book isn't a parenting book, so we're not talking about when or whether to reward your kids for things. We're simply talking about moving away from food-based rewards for the times that you do want to reward or celebrate something.

One caveat to this is that I don't think eating vegetables is something that necessarily needs a reward at all. As mundane and un-interesting a strategy as this is, just keep offering various veggies in various ways and encourage your kids to try them (and model eating them yourself). Many kids will eventually come around to them if they're not pressured or bribed. You don't need to reward their vegetable eating efforts with any type of reward – dessert or otherwise.

So what are some non-food rewards we can use with kids to either celebrate a big accomplishment (like an A+ report card) or reward other things? From small to big, here are some ideas:

- Stickers
- An extra story at bedtime
- Go to the park
- Family game night (let them choose the game)
- Family movie night (let them choose the movie)
- Extra video game time or screen time

- Bubbles or other small fun thing
- New activity book
- Art/craft supplies
- Temporary tattoos
- Play time with friends (or a sleepover if they're old enough)
- Sleepover at grandma's (a reward for parents too!)
- Let them choose a new toy from the store
- Let them choose the restaurant and go out to dinner*
- Go out to a movie
- A 1-on-1 "mommy and me" or "daddy and me" date
- Trip to the zoo
- Day at an amusement park

* I don't think going out to a restaurant is necessarily the same as eating for reward. You may not agree with that, and that's completely okay! I view it as a different location for a meal, and an enjoyable outing with loved ones. Whether at home or at a restaurant, you have to eat dinner either way, right? So yes, sometimes we eat more when we're at a restaurant, or we eat different foods than usual, but I don't see it in the same way as "going for ice cream because you did a great thing today." Of course, if you see it differently, feel free not to use this one!

Emotional Eating in Kids

Eating to deal with emotions shows up in kids younger than you may expect. Over 60% of kids ages 5-13 report eating in response to mood. Interestingly, parents of younger kids (age 2-6) report that their kids seem to *undereat* in response to stress. Some researchers believe that this is due to a change in gut motility when under stress.[46]

Therefore, it appears that eating *more* in response to stressful stimuli may be a learned behavior, and one that doesn't help us in regard to our overall health.

So how do young kids learn to eat emotionally? While it's difficult to truly determine cause and effect, there is a lot of research out there that shows correlations with both modeling (learning by example when parents eat emotionally) and controlling feeding practices (like pressuring kids to eat, using food as a reward, and/or restricting certain foods).[46,48]

"Children of mothers who use food for emotion regulation consume more sweet, palatable foods in the absence of hunger than do children of mothers who use this feeding practice infrequently. Emotional overeating behavior may occur in the context of negative mood in children whose mothers use food for emotion regulation purposes."[48] I want to point out the use of the phrase "mothers who use this feeding practice infrequently" because I am so glad they didn't draw a line in the sand to say moms who "don't" or "never" eat emotionally. As with all things when it comes to eating, no one is ever perfect!

Unfortunately, it appears that emotional eating continues and may even get worse over time as kids grow up.[46] Therefore, if we want to do what we can to prevent our kids from engaging in emotional eating both now and in the future, it's helpful to get our own emotional eating under control, and to also evaluate some of our feeding practices to be sure they're sending the message we *want* to be sending.

By eating emotionally ourselves, dealing with difficult situations with food, or using sweets as a reward, we model these behaviors for our kids to emulate. And if we're wanting to move away from doing this ourselves, it makes sense that we wouldn't want to instill emotional or reward eating in them for doing things like chores or eating their veggies.

What Else Can We Do to Prevent Emotional Eating?

Aside from working on our own example of not eating emotionally, we can help teach our kids how to regulate and manage their emotions.

1 – Help Them to Name Their Emotions

You can do this even when they're very little. When they're upset about something, see if you can pinpoint why, and name the emotion. "Oh sweetie, you're *sad* that grandma had to go home" or "I know it made you *angry* that Tyler took your toy."

2 – Find a Fix, If Possible

Just like in our own work on emotional management in the previous chapter, we can help them find a fix in the cases where one exists. In the above examples, you can't fix the fact that grandma had to go home, but you might be able to fix/address the situation with Tyler. If your child is old enough to come up with ideas on his own, see if he can think of a way to solve the problem. Maybe there are two similar toys and they can both have one, or maybe they can take turns, or maybe one kid can find something else to play with, or maybe Tyler issues an apology, etc.

3 – Non-Food Comfort

Sometimes you can't fix it, and that's okay. We can help them cope by finding ways to feel better, or helping them move on to focusing on something else. In the case of grandma going home, a hug or cuddle or some reading time might be all that's needed to help your kiddo feel better.

The basic idea is to not set the precedent of "Will a cookie help you feel better?" Any kid will likely answer that question with a yes, because just like with us, food feels like it helps at that immediate moment. But it doesn't help us learn to deal with difficult things in the long run.

Build up their emotional awareness and ability to weather the storms they come up against. They'll be armed with non-food coping mechanisms from a young age that will serve them well for life!

SECTION 6: MAINTAINING THIS NEW MINDSET

CHAPTER 18: MINDSET MAINTENANCE IN REAL LIFE

Now that we've done our mindset makeover, it's time to talk about maintaining it. If you've ever watched an actual makeover show on television (please tell me I'm not the only one who used to watch "What Not to Wear"?), then you know that the person getting the makeover usually makes a total transformation within the confines of the show.

My question, though, is always… what happens afterwards? I'm willing to bet they don't wear the same five pieces of (very expensive) clothing every day for the rest of forever, so how do they maintain their new makeover?

Hmm, that sounds rather similar to a diet, doesn't it? When a diet is over and you've perhaps lost a bit of weight (made a transformation), what happens next? Do you maintain it? Or do you revert back to your pre-diet ways?

The maintenance piece is where most diets fail. They don't give you the tools or mindset necessary to succeed in real life, and into the future. The makeover show is the same way… they give you a professional hairdresser and makeup artist, a small collection of super expensive clothes, and then send you on your way, with only a passing mention of what kinds of clothes look great on you, should you decide to buy more clothes in the future. Wow, that's not super helpful.

And that's where this makeover is different. It's not about a short-term transformation that you can't maintain. Rather, the entire point of this makeover is the maintenance piece. It's undoing the ineffectiveness of the previous diets so you can actually get the tools you need to sustain this mindset in the long term. Instead of one pair of Jimmy Choo shoes that only goes with one outfit, it's more like getting a bunch of practical and comfortable shoes that you can wear for any season and with any clothes you like. It's a very refreshing approach!

So what happens next? In order to keep this new mindset, especially in the midst of a constant onslaught of diet culture coming at you from every which way, let's talk a bit about maintenance, and how to foster and keep this mindset in our daily lives.

Your Values and Identity – Embodying This Non-Diet Approach

The first important thing to do when thinking about maintaining this new mindset, is to assess how it fits in with your identity and values. These two things are so fundamental to how we make decisions, and really, life is all about various decisions. We make bazillions of choices each day (not a true number, obviously). We don't even think about most of them!

Do I make coffee?

What should I wear today?

Do I hit "snooze" or get out of bed immediately?

Do I want to go for a run before breakfast?

What will I pack for lunch?

Which shoes will I wear?

How will I do my hair today?

Will I put on makeup?

What time should I leave to get to work?

As you read over those little decisions (all of which get made before 8:00 a.m. for many of us), you may think that the answer to some are so obvious that they're not even choices anymore. ("Do I make coffee?" Who are you kidding, of course I make coffee!) But what's profound about that is the fact that having a decision be almost on autopilot means that this thing is tied in deeply with your identity and values.

I love coffee. It makes me happy. Enjoying it with my husband as part of my morning routine is something that I look forward to every single day. I value my coffee dates with my husband. I am someone who really loves coffee.

Take special note of those last two statements. I *value* my coffee dates. I *am someone who* loves coffee. The first one speaks to my values. The second speaks to my identity. Because morning coffee is so intimately associated with one of my important values, and is something I identify as enjoying, the decision to have coffee in the morning becomes a "no-brainer."

Let's also take a non-edible example: "What will I wear today?" It's easiest to use myself as the example again, and since I've had two very different careers, I'll use both my current self and my former self to show how the same values and identity can result in different choices depending on the situation:

- **Basic info:** I value comfort, professionalism, and affordability. I am someone who wants to be respected and taken seriously at work.

- **Former self (worked in an office):** The choice of a comfortable outfit that is also appropriate and professional office wear (and likely came at a discount from Kohl's), is a no-brainer in this case. It lives my values, and fits with my identity as someone who wants to be perceived as professional and respectable.

- **Current self:** The values and identity are the same, but I now work from home and don't interact with people in person every day. My clothing choice no longer has to be something that showcases my professionalism. I tend to wear workout clothes, even if I'm not going to the gym that day, because they're comfortable and affordable.

Same values, same identity, different outcome for different situations. And it is the same way with food and eating. I value health and happiness. I value setting a healthy example for my son. I am someone who is a generally healthy person, views foods as being on a spectrum (not good or bad), and looks at the big picture of my eating.

Those values and identity color all of my eating choices. Sometimes I eat purely for the happiness and tastiness aspect of it (like a brownie, or a slice of ice cream cake). I enjoy it and it does make me happy! But I also know that if I ate those things all day, every day, I would no longer be living my value of health or my identity as a generally healthy person. So the cake and brownie are things I view in the overall spectrum of my eating and *choose* to not have them all the time, so that I can thoroughly enjoy them when I *do* decide to eat them.

Acting in Line with Your Values Can Be Its Own Reward

In the previous section, we talked about using food as a reward, and we covered some alternatives you can use in place of food. All of the things listed, however, are known as *external* rewards. They are things to enjoy that are somehow outside of ourselves. But external rewards are not the only kind of rewards. It's possible to have something be, in a sense, its own reward. It just depends on what you value.

> *"An internal or intrinsic reward is what you experience internally. It is a sense of achievement from within. It is experiencing the satisfaction that comes from your own actions."* Deepak Rajpal

I love that: "the satisfaction that comes from your own actions." By having one of our actions speak to our values in some way, we get rewarded by a deep feeling of pride or integrity. If you think about the things you do, even the ones that you may not always feel like doing in the moment, we usually have an underlying values reason. There is something about it that is important to us. I'll use some personal examples here:

- I arrive early to places because promptness is considerate of others.

- I grocery shop with my son because it exposes him to a variety of foods and experiences and sets a healthy example.

- I find ways to manage my various frustrations without food because it genuinely helps me feel better in the long run.

- I work hard on things because a solid work ethic and pride in my work are important to me.

- I recycle because I care about the planet.

- I do laundry even though I don't like to, because it's important to me that my family and I have clean clothes to wear. (And it's the same reason I wash dishes so we have clean plates to eat off, even though I hate washing dishes!)

It's totally okay to have both internal and external rewards. And yes, it's harder to think up the internal rewards; because. they're not as conducive to creating a big list like the external rewards. But that feeling of integrity that comes from acting according to the things that are important to you is actually a very powerful thing.

Take some time to think of the underlying reasons why certain things are important to you, both in general and also in terms of health choices. In what ways are some of the choices you make in those areas their own reward?

CHAPTER 19: TROUBLESHOOTING STRATEGIES FOR TOUGH SITUATIONS

Troubleshooting Part 1: Preparation

You will encounter tons of decisions each day. Some days will be easier and more routine than others; some days will be more challenging and difficult. But in maintaining this new mindset, it's helpful to see some examples of ways we can embody this approach (if it aligns with your values, of course!), especially when it comes to the tougher situations. Common decisions we'll face that will test our mindset:

- The tempting candy dish at work, or any other random tempting less-nutritious food
- The choice to exercise, or not
- Food pushers
- Social events and holidays
- Restaurant portion sizes
- Tough emotions
- Planning meals and grocery shopping

These are all incredibly common things we will make choices about as we go through our days. They may not all be difficult, but different things are tough for different people, so I thought it best to list several different examples. For all of these, and any other tough situation you find yourself in, I've come to realize that there are two approaches that work hand in hand to help you through a situation.

The first is Preparation: things we do when we're not in the immediate decision-making situation that either prevent the situation or make the situation easier.

The second is In-The-Moment: strategies you use at the time the tough situation begins, to help you make a decision you're happy about.

The Preparation part is common to just about all tough situations, so we'll cover that first, and then talk about the various In-The-Moment strategies for each of the things listed.

Preparation

When you're well rested, relaxed, and happy/content, do things feel generally easier? Think about something not food related first... like your kid making a mess with his crayons, or accidentally dumping out a whole container of toothpicks. If you're generally feeling pretty good before that happens, or you kind of anticipated that letting him carry the box of toothpicks would end up this way, you probably take it in stride, cleaning up the mess with your child in a fairly calm manner.

How does your reaction to this same situation change if you're overtired, frustrated, and already stressed out when it happens? It's harder to handle it in a way you're happy with, right? Maybe you yell at the kid, or punish him for making the mess, cleaning it up angrily by yourself while he sits in a corner. When you think back on it later when you are calmer, you realize the mess wasn't that big of a deal, and you regret yelling.

Dealing with tough food situations is the same. When we come into them already feeling well, or prepared for what we'll face, we're able to think through our response and handle it calmly . But when we're tired and cranky and caught off guard, we let our impulses get the better of us, and only think about it later.

It's for this reason that I am such an advocate for self-care. It helps us navigate all aspects of life in a calmer manner, and it allows us to stay mindful and present, even when things get tough. How do we cultivate this self-care? Rest, Joy, and Planning.

Rest

When we are overtired or fatigued, everything feels like such a daunting task. Even things we usually enjoy become just another thing on the to-do list that we don't feel like doing. It's truly amazing what getting enough sleep and allowing ourselves to rest (when we're awake) can do for us.

If you're not getting enough sleep at night, it makes everything harder. If you want to make things a bit easier on yourself, start to prioritize your sleep. On the next page there are a few things that can help:

1 – Create a Simple Bedtime Ritual

Nothing elaborate is needed here, I promise. You don't need a 30-minute bubble bath, guided meditation, and scented candles. Just a short wind-down routine to help cue your body and mind that it's time for bed.

2 – Do That Ritual at a Reasonable Time

I know none of us like to hear this, but getting to bed earlier means you'll be better rested and, therefore, better able to enjoy the following day. I know that the time after the kids go to bed is precious, believe me! And definitely do take time for yourself to enjoy the quietness of that time. But then get to bed early too, so that the next day won't feel quite so hectic and stressful. Who knows, maybe with more sleep under your belt you won't be living for the kids' bedtime the next day!

3 – Get Some Rest When You're Awake

We are always so "go-go-go" these days. We're constantly overloaded with things to do, places to go, and stuff to clean. I get it. Finding time to relax is hard! But that makes it all the more important. Find some relaxing things you enjoy doing so that you can incorporate some rest into your day. It doesn't have to take a long time. It can be as simple as listening to one 3-minute song, or reading one chapter of a book, or doodling on a piece of paper. It also doesn't have to *be* anything. Sitting on the couch, closing your eyes for a moment, and allowing yourself to do absolutely nothing for a few minutes can feel incredibly wonderful!

Joy

This ties in a little bit with the wakeful rest point above, but in that one, the goal is relaxation and rest. In this one, it's joy. Things can serve both purposes, though, in which case you've 'hit two birds with one stone,' which is pretty awesome. Coloring can be both relaxing and joyful; and the same with listening to music and reading.

The goal here is to "fill your cup." Find ways to add joy to your life. You pretty much can't go wrong with this, but it does serve two big purposes within the context we're discussing. First, adding joy to life means that we counteract some of the inevitable negative stuff that comes in. If we don't purposely add joy, it can feel like the negative things take over. And we just talked about how when we're happy, we're better able to handle tough situations in a relatively calm manner, versus when we're already unhappy.

Second, we tend to seek joy when we haven't had enough of it. Unfortunately, one of the quickest and easiest ways to inject a bit of joy is to eat something yummy, usually something sweet. When we don't have enough joy in our day, we seek it out by turning to food, and that's not usually something we feel good about afterwards. So purposely adding non-food joy to our day helps to prevent us turning to food for non-hunger or emotional reasons.

Planning

There will always be situations that catch us off guard, but there are also tons of tough situations that we know about ahead of time. Making a tentative plan for those situations can be a huge help in navigating them in a way we're happy with. It allows us to think through the decision logically, when we're not *in* the moment. There is even a psychological theory called "Decision Fatigue" which explains that the more decisions we have to make each day, the more our will power and self-control become depleted, making it harder and harder to make more good decisions. For this reason, I love the idea of pre-deciding as many things in our day as we can. Remember the little decisions I mentioned earlier, like "Will I make coffee?" or "What will I wear today?" If we can decide those things ahead of time by pre-deciding, then when the time comes, we don't deplete our mental resources by needing to make a new decision each time. This leaves us open and available to make other, more difficult decisions later on.

In trying to pre-decide a plan for a situation that I know is looming, one of my favorite ways of approaching it is to ask myself "What choice will leave me feeling proud of myself afterwards?"

I think I mentioned this in the Good/Bad Foods section too. It's something I use when I'm going somewhere that I know will have loads of dessert options. I know they'll all probably look yummy, and I don't want to say "no" to all of them, but I also don't want to *eat* all of them! So I plan ahead to think about how I can feel proud of myself afterwards. That usually, for me, means trying a very small piece of the two or three things that look best. Or it might mean scoping out only the best-looking dessert and having just that one. In both cases, I still prioritize the more nutritious foods before I get to the desserts, so I live my values of eating generally healthy and keeping the less-nutritious food a small part of the bigger picture. But pre-deciding how I want to handle the desserts makes it easier to navigate that situation once I'm in it.

Troubleshooting 2: Specific Strategies

Okay, let's dive in to some strategies that you can use for these common, tough situations…

1 – Tempting Treats

We now know that these aren't "bad" foods. But since they are less nutritious than many other choices, and we value our overall health, it makes sense to not eat every single one we see. When you're tempted by the latest yummy-looking treat, for which you didn't have a chance to pre-decide, it's helpful to give yourself some sort of pause to think through the choice.

It's much more enjoyable and empowering, to choose to eat it because you consciously decided to, not because your hand popped it in your mouth faster than your mind could catch up. We don't tend to regret the choices we make to enjoy something yummy. We do sometimes regret the ones that happened without a single thought. So the idea is to pause long enough to make a decision that you truly want to make. Some questions you can ask yourself at times like these:

- Am I actually legitimately hungry? If so, should I eat some more nutritious food first and have this with my meal?
- Is this something I can take now and save to eat later if I still want it?

- Do I actually really enjoy this thing, or would I be eating it just because it's there?

- Have I eaten a lot of similar things lately and can maybe pass this one up?

These may or may not speak to you, so feel free to come up with your own. The general premise behind them is to determine if it's something that would be actually enjoyed; if it has to be enjoyed now or can it wait until later; and if there have already been lots of these types of foods eaten recently, they might be crowding out some more-nutritious food.

2 – The Choice to Exercise, or Not

I'm going to preface this with the fact that I am not a trainer, nor am I an expert in exercise science. I just want to share what works for me and has also worked for my clients.

When it comes to fitting in exercise, I find that the preparation stage is crucial. If my workout is planned/scheduled, my clothes are ready to go, and I have a solid idea of why I want to exercise, it is much more likely to actually happen. Sometimes that preparation part is all we really need, especially if our values and identity are also closely tied to movement we enjoy!

However, I think we all have days when we just don't feel like it. Sometimes our bodies are telling us that we need more rest; in which case, I tend to think it's wise to listen (which comes back to the Preparation piece I spoke about earlier... getting enough rest so that everything else is easier!).

Other times, we just don't feel like it in the moment. When that happens, I find it helpful to ask two questions:

1. What is my goal with the exercise/workout/movement I planned to do today?
2. How important is that to me?

This helps remind me why I'm doing this in the first place. With my aerial practice, if I'm working toward a performance piece, I have a clear goal that is important to me. If I'm not, it can feel easier to skip it, even though improving my skills in general is still important to me.

If I'm still on the fence after remembering that something is important to me, then I ask myself if I can do just five minutes. Many times, if I just start, I end up doing more than the five minutes, or even finishing a whole workout or class. Lower the bar so it doesn't feel so daunting. Once you start, you might get back into the "mood" for it. (Thanks, endorphins!)

3- Food Pushers

We know who some of them are. We all have a relative who, at every family gathering, is always trying to put more things on your plate. Sometimes it's more than one relative too! Food pushers are everywhere: "Try this!"— "Have more of that!"— "Why aren't you eating?"— Etc., etc., etc.

When we don't know the person, it's easier to say no to food we don't want to eat. But when it's a loved one and you fear hurting their feelings, saying no feels harder. The basic idea in getting through it is to honor your preferences and values, which includes your value of not offending loved ones! So how do we strike that balance? Sometimes it's all in how you say something.

- "That looks delicious, but I'm so full already. Thanks, though!"
- "I'm not hungry now, but that looks amazing. Can I take some for later?"
- "No thanks, I'm good for now."

These are some examples of ways you can politely say no and still keep the person's feelings intact. You don't want to say, "That looks gross, I'm not eating that!" So tell them it seems delightful but that you're either not hungry, or already full, or are just "good for now, maybe later, though." They may still push, but stand your ground.

4 – Social Events and Holidays

Strategies here are a compilation of the ones already mentioned… planning ahead and handling food pushers. Holidays tend to have lots of food, lots of drinks and desserts, and lots of people telling you to try the thing they brought to the party.

The best way to tackle these situations is to plan ahead and do as much pre-deciding as possible. You usually know how most of these events will go… the food that will be there, the desserts that people will bring, etc. So ask yourself that question: "What choices will make me feel proud afterwards?" and then politely handle the food pushers once you get there!

5 – Restaurant Portion Sizes

When we're at home, it's relatively easy to serve ourselves an amount that we're likely to eat. When we go out to eat, though, we don't know what the portion sizes will be. Restaurants are notorious for giving one person enough food to feed an army. That wouldn't seem like a bad thing if it wasn't for the fact that it makes it super hard for us to stop before we're stuffed.

If you're going to be going out to eat, there are a few strategies you can employ to keep your healthy eating values and your tummy comfort in mind. I mentioned some of these in the section on the Clean Plate Club, but here are some other ideas too.

First, awareness always helps. Just remembering that the portions are usually ridiculous can help us remember that we don't have to eat it all.

Second, as always, go in with a plan. If you're able to look up the menu ahead of time, you can pre-decide what you're having. That is a bonus for people like me who take forever to make a decision on what to order! You have time to really look over the options, and make a choice you'll be happy with. Also, if you have a say in the restaurant choice, you can always propose ones where you know there are some healthier and appropriately sized options.

Don't assume you need to get a full meal. Since appetizers also tend to be large, getting one of those and a side of veggies or salad can be a really lovely, just-the-right-size meal. Not to mention, it's often cheaper! (Remember, one of my values is affordability!)

If you do get a full meal, look it over when it arrives. Is this enough for two meals? If so, get a to-go box right away and put half away for tomorrow's lunch. The extra won't be staring you in the face to tempt you, and you've got tomorrow's lunch taken care of. Win!

If it's not quite enough for another full meal, see if you can estimate how much you'd eat if you were home and this meal was on your typical plate. Have you ever taken home leftovers, put them on a plate, and thought they grew in size? It's because restaurants tend to use odd plates, and theirs are often much bigger than regular household ones, making the huge size of the meal not quite so obvious. It's tough to estimate how some things translate to your household plates, but give it your best guess. Then stop when you reach the point you think you'd have stopped at home. You can box up the rest, or toss it depending on how much is left (or share with your dining companions!).

I'm always a fan of splitting dinner. Now, this doesn't work with my husband, since he can usually eat an entire entrée plus some of mine. But with someone else who eats around the same amount, and has the same tastes that you do, it can be a nice way to keep the meal affordable and appropriately portioned. Even if I don't split a meal, I almost always split dessert, if I get it at all.

Another quick tip for dealing with these big portions: slow down your eating. We often plow right through, only realizing after the plate is clean that we're over-stuffed. If we slow down, we can periodically tune in and see if we're already satisfied before we become uncomfortable.

6 – Tough Emotions

There was an entire section on this, so I won't reiterate everything here. The name of the game is to be aware of the times when we tend to turn to food or drinks in order to manage our emotions. Our desire to turn to food tells us that we're uncomfortable with being uncomfortable, and that perhaps we don't have enough other coping strategies at our disposal.

Mindfulness is important here (as it usually is). Be mindful of the urge to turn to food, and remember that we don't have to act on our urges when they're not helpful to us in the long run (like punching your boss when he's a jerk… we don't want to get fired!). Here's the graphic again, to help you remember the various options you have when you're facing a negative feeling.

Response Options to Negative Emotions

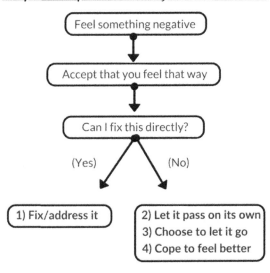

7 – Planning Meals and Grocery Shopping

This isn't a "tricky situation" per se, since it's something many of us do each week. But it is something that really either helps or hinders our decision-making on a daily basis. If you want to make more nutritious choices more often than not, planning ahead for healthy and nourishing meals is a big part of the puzzle. (There we go with the pre-deciding again!)

When planning for healthy and nutritious meals, produce is king. Be sure to include a variety of fruits and vegetables that you and your family enjoy; then round it out with protein, carbohydrate, and fat sources. There will usually be some less-nutritious foods included on your list each week, and that's completely okay. But try to take a birds-eye view and have the nutritious stuff outweigh the less-nutritious stuff.

When shopping, we almost inevitably pass by some type of tempting food that's not on our list. Sometimes that tempting thing is also nutritious, and sometimes it's not. This is where your in-the-moment skills come into play in similar fashion to any other temptation. Questions to ask yourself:

- Is this something I (or my family) really enjoy or would be really interested in trying?
- Do we have lots of other less-nutritious items planned this week? If so, can we swap one to make room for this one if we prefer this one?
- Will this same item be available next time I'm at the store, so I can get it then if I don't get it now?

The same general themes apply: how the food fits into the bigger picture, and if it's possible to wait. Some things are "limited edition" or seasonal and really aren't around all the time (like pumpkin spiced *everything*, once September hits). In that case, perhaps the thing you're eyeing really won't be around next time, so if you want to try it, get it now. You can always swap out something else you'd planned for.

Again, the thing to keep in mind is that you don't have to say "yes" to every less-nutritious tempting food opportunity, nor do you need to always say "no." It's about the overall picture. Plan a majority of nutritious foods, and then sprinkle in the other foods in a way that works for you and your family.

CHAPTER 20: FIGHTING BACK AGAINST SOCIETY'S DIET CULTURE

Part of maintaining this non-diet mindset is being able to resist the diet culture that is all around us. As we mentioned in the body image section, everything is marketed to women by creating or pointing out "flaws" that can only be fixed by the product or service being sold. We are constantly told we are not good enough as we are. Not only that, but the focus on looks – from the media, from society as a whole, from comments from the people around us – is so deep-rooted in our society that it's hard to get away from it.

While we're probably not going to overhaul society's collective diet- and beauty-centered thinking in the near future, it's still a worthy endeavor to pick it apart whenever we get the chance. Sometimes, an alternate viewpoint is just what others need to hear.

Remember to Take the Focus Off Looks and Weight

One way that we can start to spread this new viewpoint is something I mentioned in the body image section: stop commenting on other people's looks. Yes, this is usually subtle. Someone may not even notice that you didn't compliment their weight loss, or their complexion, or how pretty they are. But you can start to shift the focus away from those things and onto things that matter so much more.

Finding non-beauty things to comment on is tough at first, especially when you're just starting. I'm fairly new at it too, and I catch myself all the time. But it's amazing how it opens your eyes to seeing things on a deeper level than just skin-deep. It reminds us that we're all just human, and seeing the whole person instead of just their looks makes life a bit more interesting.

The Exception to This Idea

I want to say that I don't think we need to try to pretend like we're blind. We do use our eyes, and it's very hard to pretend like we don't see something, especially if it's something we want to compliment. So here is how I attempt to draw a distinction... I try not to comment on a person's body size or shape, or make assumptions based on what I see.

Sometimes a person makes a sudden and noticeable (voluntary) change, like getting their hair cut or colored, or they get a new tattoo, or pierce their ears. We tend to notice those things, and I don't think complimenting those things is a bad idea. We're not commenting on the person or their body as a whole, we're commenting on a specific, noticeable change: "I like your new hair color!" or "What a cool tattoo!"

Where things start to get questionable is when we comment on the general size, shape, or state of someone's body. And while I think most of us are kind enough to know that commenting on someone's weight gain isn't usually a nice idea, we tend to have no problem complimenting someone's weight loss, or thinness.

I know that I've done this myself. We see that someone has lost weight and we want to compliment it. Many of us tend to default to a general "You lost weight! You look great!" comment. And while that's meant in the nicest way possible, there can be a small hint of comparison there… suggesting that the new smaller version is "great" and the previous heavier version was not.

We actually make a lot of assumptions about weight loss in other people. We assume that they wanted to lose weight. We assume they are healthier now. We assume they're happier now. We assume they did it in a way that wasn't a completely horrible experience. We assume they're happy with their new body size/shape.

But we don't actually know the whole story, do we? We don't know if they have a medical condition that resulted in quick weight loss and actually means they're very sick. We don't know if they starved themselves and suffered tremendously to lose this weight. We don't know if they are any healthier or happier than they were before. We do not know what "baggage" has come along with this weight loss that our eyes can't see.

The same idea goes for someone's general thinness. We assume a lot of things about people who seem to be naturally thin, or have just always been thin in the time we've known them. But again, we never know the whole story. We don't know if someone is actually suffering with an eating disorder, or significant body image issues, or if they're actually very sick.

So, while I absolutely and completely understand the desire to comment on someone's weight loss, I think it's still something better left unsaid. Our eyes can't know the whole story, and commenting on weight, even when it's complimentary, can be very uncomfortable for many people.

So the moral of this story is: don't comment on a person's weight or general looks. While these comments and compliments usually come from a kind-hearted place, they include a lot of assumptions, and we don't know how our comments might affect the person's mindset, or that of anyone else listening to the conversation. It also perpetuates the underlying idea that being thin or losing weight is "good" and being large, or gaining weight is "bad." And those assumptions are simply not true.

What Can We Do Instead?

I know, this is really hard to wrap our brains around, isn't it? We're so used to saying these things in the spirit of being nice and making conversation. If we shouldn't be talking about this, what should we talk about?

Ask about the *person*. Don't comment on weight or size, just ask how they're doing, and what's new in their world. They might choose to talk about work, or their kids, or their upcoming vacation, or maybe they will bring up their weight loss and say how thrilled they are with it. If they do, a simple "I'm so happy for you" is a kind reply that doesn't further the weight conversation. And of course, if they don't bring it up, keep chatting about whatever else they are interested in talking about!

Helping Others Reframe Their Comments

Oh boy, this one can be a touchy subject! None of us wants to be that person who always corrects the people around them. That gets annoying pretty fast. But every once in a while, it can help to shine a bit of light on how unintentionally judgmental a comment can be.

Reframing comments from others, in as polite a way as possible, is another great way we can start to fight back against this culture. Have you ever been with someone and they made a rude comment to you about someone else's appearance? Or perhaps their own? It's an uncomfortable situation for sure. But in the spirit of trying to spread this idea of compassion around, I'm starting to speak up.

When someone comments on another person's body or how they look, I'll say something about how we don't know the person's whole story. Or I'll comment positively on some other aspect of the person if I can, or if I know them. If I'm comfortable enough with the person who said the comment, I'll actually gently call them out on it by telling them the comment they made wasn't very nice.

I also try to help people reframe their comments about themselves. We have a tendency to be pretty self-deprecating, and for some reason, it's actually seen as socially acceptable or common to say negative things about ourselves. Perhaps because we're trying a bit too hard to not come across as boastful or narcissistic? I don't know.

What's particularly sad is that we're usually even more self-defeating in our minds than what comes out of our mouths. We censor it a bit, or say it in a half-joking manner when we talk negatively about ourselves to others. But I know that when I hear someone talk negatively about themselves, they probably feel even *more* negatively about it than they're actually saying. And I want to do my best to change that.

It's tough, of course, to find the balance between honestly and genuinely helping, and coming across as patronizing. But I try to keep three things in mind (which will sound pretty familiar after the Body Image section):

1 – Acceptance

2 – Compassion

3 – Growth mindset

Friends and loved ones are the people most likely to air their self-negativity to you at some point, and one of the kindest things you can do is help them reframe that negativity into the above ideas. Acknowledge what they're feeling, and don't dwell on the negativity. Tell them how a person's body size/shape/weight honestly doesn't matter. It's not important. What is more important is how they feel, both physically and mentally. Steer the conversation to how you can help them, and how they're not stuck with whatever it is they're upset about.

Believing that we can change, and coming to it from a place of acceptance is something foreign to many of us, and we need a helping hand to get there. Be that helping hand for the people you care about, and spread these ideas to them so that they can start fighting back against society's body-shaming nonsense too.

Social Media

Oh man, social media. It's such a blessing and also a curse. On one hand, we can more easily keep in touch with friends and family who aren't nearby. On the other hand, it allows us to see all sorts of crazy articles and things being shared from people we only barely know, or who are friends of friends. I can't even count the number of diet culture, detox, ate-it-now-negate-it, fat-shaming, pseudo-science things I've come across on Facebook. It's incredibly disheartening. And it is everywhere! So again, we try to do our part, little by little, to fight back.

- If you see something blatantly body-shaming being shared, speak up about how it's not okay.
- If you see a rare gem of body-positive information being posted, share it!
- For every piece of pseudo-science you come across, share something that actually promotes the truth.
- Engage in conversations and polite debates if you have the time (and can stand it). This is something I have a difficult time with myself, but it's something I want to get better about.
- If someone on your friends list constantly shares this negative stuff, feel free to unfriend or unfollow them!

Social media is a place where we can end up being bombarded by diet culture. We can't stop it from being out there, but we can stop sharing it, and we can start sharing the opposite viewpoint. You never know how many of your friends will start to read the more positive and compassionate things you share and start to view the world in a similar way. What this entire section comes down to is this idea: "Be the change you wish to see in the world." It's hard, yes, but so very important to spread positivity, acceptance, and kindness in a world that seems to be constantly pulled down by negativity.

CHAPTER 21: CONSISTENTLY INSTILLING THIS MINDSET IN OUR KIDS

If we've learned one thing throughout this book in terms of kids, it's that they learn tremendously by our example. When our behaviors and actions stem from a diet mindset, and we're always talking negatively about our bodies, or saying how bad certain foods are, or constantly stepping on the scale and counting our calories, it sends a message... one we usually don't want to send.

So as I've said in several places, the first thing we can do to set our kids up for non-diet success is to stop dieting ourselves, and to do this mindset makeover. How they approach food and eating starts with us, first and foremost. Of course, there are ways we can help to guide them in this direction as well, besides just our example. This chapter is essentially a summary of the important points from each of the kid-specific chapters in the book, so that you have a quick reference place for the overall idea of how I like to approach this mindset with kids, and the things we can do to help instill it in them so they grow up with a healthy food relationship.

Consistently Instill a Positive Body Image in Them

- Focus and comment on what their bodies can do, not how they look.
- Appreciate those things.
- Be sure they know that they are loved and worthy and valuable exactly as they are.
- Teach them that how their body looks is only one very small piece of who they are.
- Teach them to care for their body because their body deserves to be treated kindly.
- Model and teach healthy behaviors as a way to care for their bodies.
- When they're older, help them become aware of the unrealistic standards all around us.

Help Them to Eat Well Without Viewing Foods as Good or Bad

- Provide a variety of foods, with most of them being nutritious.
- Provide a consistent, yet flexible, structure for meals and snacks.
- Don't use bribes or rewards to get them to eat veggies.

Help Them Find a Balanced Approach to Managing Sweets

- Don't let "because it's bad for you" be a reason not to eat something.

- Create your boundaries for the less-nutritious foods, and help them stick to them.
- If you have to say no to something, tell them why, and when they'll get something similar next.

Guide Them to Eat According to Their Hunger and Fullness Signals

- Use a meal and snack structure to avoid grazing and encourage development of hunger.
- Let them eat until they're satisfied, even if it seems like a lot.
- If they're not hungry, don't force them to eat.
- Remind them how long it will be until the next meal/snack.
- Watch for "taste hunger" and balance it by using your goodies boundaries.

Help Them Understand and Manage Their Emotions

- Acknowledge and name their feelings. Help them fix the problem, if possible, and have them contribute ideas for how to fix it.
- Give non-food comfort when you can't fix it.

Keep an Open Dialogue About Health, Bodies, and Eating

- When they have questions about food, bodies, or eating, answer honestly (and age-appropriately)
- When kids are old enough, point out how advertisements tell us we have "problems" to "fix."
- Point out unrealistic media images.

- Speak kindly of others, focusing on things other than looks and weight.
- Encourage acceptance, appreciation, kindness, and compassion in themselves and others.

CONCLUSION

I want to thank you for reading this book. It was a labor of love, and if it helped you to start moving away from a dieting mindset, even just a little bit, I am so very thrilled. I wish we could magically instill a healthy and happy food relationship into every person on the planet, but since it doesn't work that way, I hope that you will share what you've learned here with your friends and loved ones. Loan them your book, or recommend it the next time someone mentions the latest juice cleanse they've decided to try. Do your part to spread compassion and kindness, since so many people are out there spending incredible amounts of time and energy disliking themselves and their bodies. Embody this non-diet mindset, and see how much freer and calmer you feel about food and eating!

REFERENCES

1. Goldstein SP, Katterman SN, Lowe MR. Relationship of dieting and restrained eating to self-reported caloric intake in female college freshmen. Eat Behav. 2013;14(2):237-240. doi:10.1016/j.eatbeh.2012.12.002.
2. de Witt Huberts JC, Evers C, de Ridder DTD. Double trouble: restrained eaters do not eat less and feel worse. Psychol Health. 2013;28(6):686-700. doi:10.1080/08870446.2012.751106.
3. De Ridder D, Adriaanse M, Evers C, Verhoeven A. Who diets? Most people and especially when they worry about food. Appetite. 2014;80:103-108. doi:10.1016/j.appet.2014.05.011.
4. Lowe MR, Doshi SD, Katterman SN, Feig EH, Avena N, Barbarich-Marsteller NC. Dieting and restrained eating as prospective predictors of weight gain. 2013. doi:10.3389/fpsyg.2013.00577.
5. Andrés A, Saldaña C. Body dissatisfaction and dietary restraint influence binge eating behavior. Nutr Res. 2014;34(11):944-950. doi:10.1016/j.nutres.2014.09.003.
6. Lowe MR, Annunziato RA, Markowitz JT, et al. Multiple types of dieting prospectively predict weight gain during the freshman year of college. Appetite. 2006;47(1):83-90. doi:10.1016/j.appet.2006.03.160.
7. Neumark-Sztainer D, Wall M, Guo J, Story M, Haines J, Eisenberg M. Obesity, disordered eating, and eating disorders in a longitudinal study of adolescents: How do dieters fare 5 years later? J Am Diet Assoc. 2006;106(4):559-568. doi:10.1016/j.jada.2006.01.003.
8. Hart KE, Chiovari P. Inhibition of eating behavior: Negative cognitive effects of dieting. J Clin Psychol. 1998;54(4):427-430. doi:10.1002/(SICI)1097-4679(199806)54:4<427::AID-JCLP4>3.0.CO;2-K.
9. Lowe MR, Levine AS. Eating Motives and the Controversy over Dieting: Eating Less Than Needed versus Less Than Wanted. Obes Res. 2005;13(5):797-806. doi:10.1038/oby.2005.90.
10. Massey A, Hill AJ. Dieting and food craving. A descriptive, quasi-prospective study. Appetite. 2012;58(3):781-785. doi:10.1016/j.appet.2012.01.020.
11. Kuijer RG, Boyce JA. Chocolate cake. Guilt or celebration? Associations with healthy eating attitudes, perceived behavioural control, intentions and weight-loss. Appetite. 2014;74:48-54. doi:10.1016/j.appet.2013.11.013.
12. Satter E. Your Child's Weight: Helping Without Harming. Kelcy Press; 2005.
13. Spiel EC, Paxton SJ, Yager Z. Weight attitudes in 3- to 5-year-old children: Age differences and cross-sectional predictors. Body Image. 2012;9(4):524-527. doi:10.1016/j.bodyim.2012.07.006.
14. Perez M, Kroon Van Diest AM, Smith H, Sladek MR. Body Dissatisfaction and Its Correlates in 5- to 7-Year-Old Girls: A Social Learning Experiment. J Clin Child Adolesc Psychol. June 2016:1-13. doi:10.1080/15374416.2016.1157758.
15. Lowes J, Tiggemann M. Body dissatisfaction, dieting awareness and the impact of parental influence in young children. Br J Health Psychol. 2003;8(2):135-147. doi:10.1348/135910703321649123.
16. Evans EH, Adamson AJ, Basterfield L, et al. Risk factors for eating disorder symptoms at 12 years of age: A 6-year longitudinal cohort study. Appetite. 2017;108:12-20. doi:10.1016/j.appet.2016.09.005.

17. Tatangelo G, McCabe M, Mellor D, Mealey A. A systematic review of body dissatisfaction and sociocultural messages related to the body among preschool children. Body Image. 2016;18:86-95. doi:10.1016/j.bodyim.2016.06.003.
18. Golden NH, Schneider M, Wood C. Preventing Obesity and Eating Disorders in Adolescents. 2016;138(3). doi:10.1542/peds.2016-1649.
19. Martini MCS, Assumpção D de, Barros MB de A, et al. Are normal-weight adolescents satisfied with their weight? Sao Paulo Med J. 2016;134(3):219-227. doi:10.1590/1516-3180.2015.01850912.
20. Sutin AR, Terracciano A. Body Weight Misperception in Adolescence and Incident Obesity in Young Adulthood. Psychol Sci. 2015;26(4):507-511. doi:10.1177/0956797614566319.
21. Cuypers K, Kvaløy K, Bratberg G, et al. Being Normal Weight but Feeling Overweight in Adolescence May Affect Weight Development into Young Adulthood—An 11-Year Followup: The HUNT Study, Norway. J Obes. 2012;2012:1-8. doi:10.1155/2012/601872.
22. Rodgers RF, Wertheim EH, Damiano SR, Gregg KJ, Paxton SJ. Stop eating lollies and do lots of sports: a prospective qualitative study of the development of children's awareness of dietary restraint and exercise to lose weight. Int J Behav Nutr Phys Act. 2015;12:155. doi:10.1186/s12966-015-0318-x.
23. Rolland K, Farnill D, Griffiths RA. Body figure perceptions and eating attitudes among Australian schoolchildren aged 8 to 12 years. Int J Eat Disord. 1997;21(3):273-278. http://www.ncbi.nlm.nih.gov/pubmed/9097200. Accessed July 25, 2017.
24. Jacobsen M. Eating Disorder Prevention (Part 1): 3 Things Every Parent Must Know - Maryann Jacobsen. http://www.maryannjacobsen.com/2010/03/eating-disorder-prevention-part-1-3-things-every-parent-must-know/. Published 2010. Accessed June 2, 2017.
25. Eaton DK, Kann L, Kinchen S, et al. Youth risk behavior surveillance - United States, 2011. MMWR Surveill Summ. 2012;61(4):1-162. http://www.ncbi.nlm.nih.gov/pubmed/22673000. Accessed June 2, 2017.
26. Lampard AM, Maclehose RF, Eisenberg ME, Neumark-Sztainer D, Davison KK, Lampard A. Weight-related Teasing in the School Environment: Associations with Psychosocial Health and Weight Control Practices among Adolescent Boys and Girls. J Youth Adolesc. 2014;43(10):1770-1780. doi:10.1007/s10964-013-0086-3.
27. van den Berg PA, Keery H, Eisenberg M, Neumark-Sztainer D, van den Berg P. Maternal and Adolescent Report of Mothers' Weight-Related Concerns and Behaviors: Longitudinal Associations with Adolescent Body Dissatisfaction and Weight Control Practices. doi:10.1093/jpepsy/jsq042.
28. Coffman DL, Balantekin KN, Savage JS. Using Propensity Score Methods To Assess Causal Effects of Mothers' Dieting Behavior on Daughters' Early Dieting Behavior. Child Obes. 2016;12(5):334-340. doi:10.1089/chi.2015.0249.
29. Neumark-Sztainer D, Bauer KW, Friend S, Hannan PJ, Story M, Berge JM. Family weight talk and dieting: how much do they matter for body dissatisfaction and disordered eating behaviors in adolescent girls? J Adolesc Health. 2010;47(3):270-276. doi:10.1016/j.jadohealth.2010.02.001.
30. Hillard EE, Gondoli DM, Corning AF, Morrissey RA. In it together: Mother talk of weight concerns moderates negative outcomes of encouragement to lose weight on daughter body dissatisfaction and disordered eating. Body Image. 2016;16:21-27. doi:10.1016/j.bodyim.2015.09.004.
31. Loth K, Fulkerson JA, Neumark-Sztainer D. Food-related parenting practices and child and adolescent weight and weight-related behaviors. Clin Pract (Lond). 2014;11(2):207-220. doi:10.2217/cpr.14.5.

32. Stevens H. Stop telling your friends they're beautiful — it's making them sick. Chicago Tribune. http://www.chicagotribune.com/lifestyles/stevens/ct-beauty-sick-stop-complimenting-women-balancing-0424-20170424-column.html. Published 2017. Accessed October 6, 2017.

33. Khazan O, Neff K. Why Self Compassion Works Better Than Self-Esteem - The Atlantic. https://www.theatlantic.com/health/archive/2016/05/why-self-compassion-works-better-than-self-esteem/481473/. Accessed June 19, 2017.

34. Neff K. Why We Should Stop Chasing Self-Esteem and Start Developing Self-Compassion. http://self-compassion.org/why-we-should-stop-chasing-self-esteem-and-start-developing-self-compassion/. Accessed June 19, 2017.

35. Hall P, Meule A, Mantzios M, Egan HH. On the Role of Self-compassion and Self-kindness in Weight Regulation and Health Behavior Change. Front Psychol Front Psychol. 2017;8(8):2293389-229. doi:10.3389/fpsyg.2017.00229.

36. Neff K. What Self-Compassion is Not: self-esteem, self-pity, indulgence. http://self-compassion.org/what-self-compassion-is-not-2/. Accessed July 28, 2017.

37. Jacobsen M. How to Raise a Mindful Eater. RMI Books; 2016.

38. Palascha A, van Kleef E, van Trijp HC. How does thinking in Black and White terms relate to eating behavior and weight regain? J Health Psychol. 2015;20(5):638-648. doi:10.1177/1359105315573440.

39. Byrne SM, Cooper Z, Fairburn CG. Psychological predictors of weight regain in obesity. Behav Res Ther. 2004;42(11):1341-1356. doi:10.1016/j.brat.2003.09.004.

40. Meule A, Westenh??fer J, K??bler A. Food cravings mediate the relationship between rigid, but not flexible, control of eating behavior and dieting success. Appetite. 2011;57(3):582-584. doi:10.1016/j.appet.2011.07.013.

41. Sairanen E, Lappalainen R, Lapveteläinen A, Tolvanen A, Karhunen L. Flexibility in weight management. Eat Behav. 2014;15(2):218-224. doi:10.1016/j.eatbeh.2014.01.008.

42. Tarrasch R, Margalit-Shalom L, Berger R. Enhancing Visual Perception and Motor Accuracy among School Children through a Mindfulness and Compassion Program. Front Psychol. 2017;8(February):1-10. doi:10.3389/fpsyg.2017.00281.

43. Dr. Dina Rose. How Parents Teach Kids to Lie About Hunger- It's Not About Nutrition. http://itsnotaboutnutrition.com/2014/07/17/how-parents-teach-kids-to-lie-about-hunger/. Accessed August 16, 2017.

44. Heatherton TF, Baumeister RF. Binge eating as escape from self-awareness. Psychol Bull. 1991;110(1):86-108. doi:10.1037/0033-2909.110.1.86.

45. Evers C, Marijn Stok F, de Ridder DTD. Feeding your feelings: emotion regulation strategies and emotional eating. Personal Soc Psychol Bull. 2010;36(6):792-804. doi:10.1177/0146167210371383.

46. Farrow C V., Haycraft E, Blissett JM. Teaching our children when to eat: how parental feeding practices inform the development of emotional eating--a longitudinal experimental design. Am J Clin Nutr. 2015;101(5):908-913. doi:10.3945/ajcn.114.103713.

47. Stinson A. Why Using Food As A Reward Is Bad For You. Elite Daily. https://www.elitedaily.com/wellness/dangers-using-food-reward-according-psychotherapist/1987373. Published 2017. Accessed January 1, 2017.

48. Blissett J, Haycraft E, Farrow C. Inducing preschool children's emotional eating: relations with parental feeding practices. Am J Clin Nutr. 2010;92(2):359-365. doi:10.3945/ajcn.2010.29375.

49. Weisenberger J. Say "Yes!" to Non-Food Rewards. http://www.eatright.org/resource/health/wellness/healthy-aging/say-yes-to-non-food-rewards. Published 2017. Accessed June 23, 2017.

50. Castle J. Why it's a bad idea to use food as a reward. https://www.bundoo.com/articles/why-its-a-bad-idea-to-use-food-as-a-reward/. Accessed June 23, 2017.

51. Lu J, Xiong S, Arora N, Dub? L. Using food as reinforcer to shape children's non-food behavior: The adverse nutritional effect doubly moderated by reward sensitivity and gender. Eat Behav. 2015;19:94-97. doi:10.1016/j.eatbeh.2015.07.003.

ABOUT THE AUTHOR

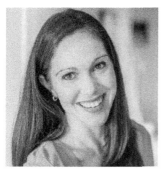

Kara Beutel is a former Nutrition Coach with a Master's of Science in Nutrition and a Bachelor's Degree in Chemistry. In her years as a coach with Georgie Fear's company One By One Nutrition, she worked with clients to repair their relationship with food and learn healthy eating habits so they could eat well without dieting. The approach focuses on small, manageable changes so that clients feel successful and empowered, and know they are capable of eating well no matter what the reality of their life looks like.

If you're interested in more personalized help repairing your relationship with food, and learning how to eat well for life without resorting to diet rules, please seek out Georgie Fear at her website GeorgieFear.com. She is a true expert in this field, and her guidance and coaching are worth their weight in diamonds!

Made in the USA
Columbia, SC
27 April 2020